Bedside Paediatrics

Sultan Mustafa

Professor and Head of Department, Paediatrics and Neonatology.
Karachi Medical and Dental College and
Abbasi Shaheed Hospital, Karachi

Sumbal Waheed

Senior Registrar, Department of Paediatrics
Karachi Medical and Dental College and
Abbasi Shaheed Hospital, Karachi

Paramount Books (Pvt.) Ltd.

Karachi | Lahore | Islamabad | Sukkur | Faisalabad | Peshawar | Abbottabad

© **Paramount** Books (Pvt.) Ltd.

Bedside Paediatrics

by

Sultan Mustafa/Sumbal Waheed

First Edition 2008
Second Edition................................2014
Third Edition 2016

Paramount Books (Pvt.) Ltd.

152/O, Block-2, P.E.C.H.S., Karachi-75400. Tel: 34310030
Fax: 34553772, E-mail: info@paramountbooks.com.pk
Website: www.paramountbooks.com.pk

ISBN: 978-969-637-175-5
Printed in Pakistan

Contents

Dedicated to

My parents

and

My children

Mustafa, Waheed and Shahana

Preface to First Edition

It is a great pleasure for me to introduce the first edition of 'Bedside Paediatrics'. I have tried my level best to write this book in such a way, that it will be comprehensible to undergraduate and postgraduate students.

There are 23 chapters in this book including chapters on ECG, CXR, paediatric procedure, paediatric formulas and normal laboratory data. Every chapter of the book has been carefully scrutinized for possible improvement.

Hats off to many of my past and present colleagues, friends and well-wishers for lots of goodwill, ideas and cooperation, Prof Syed Inkisar Ali, Dr Shamsa Farooqui, Dr Khawaja Habibi, Dr Madiha, Dr Ali, Dr Muhammad Arif, Dr Shamim Ashraf, Dr Qazi Salman and Dr Rehman deserve a special mention. All of us have worked hard to produce an edition that will be helpful to those who provide care for children and desire more about children.

Professor Ghaffar Billoo, has been kind and gracious enough to guide me and offer his invaluable advice in the preparation of the manuscript, proofreading and writing the foreword inspite of his busy schedule. I am deeply indebted to him for bestowing this honour upon me.

I hope this book, by virtue of its simplicity will prove and establish itself as a recognised book of paediatrics.

Karachi, Pakistan
April, 2008

Sultan Mustafa
MBBS, MCPS, FCPS
Associate Professor and Head
Department of Paediatrics, KM&DC and ASH

Preface to Third Edition

It is my pleasure to introduce the third edition of 'Bedside Paediatrics'. I put my maximum efforts to make it a paragon of knowledge but the chances of human error are always there, so I repent and regret any inadvertent, fortuitous or incidental shortcoming. I always welcome the criticism, suggestions and feedback from the reader.

I am thankful to Allah, Who blessed me with such competence throughout this destiny and venture. Hats off to my mother who always implores blessing for me from Allah, and my wife for her continued support and encouragement not only in this endeavour but in my whole life.

I am really thankful to my colleagues, friends and well my wishers for all goodwill and cooperation.

I hope, this book 'Bedside Paediatrics' will establish itself as a standard book of Paediatrics for undergraduates and post graduates-Inshallah.

Prof Sultan Mustafa

April, 2016

Acknowledgements

Grateful acknowledgements are made for permission to use/adopt/ reproduce certain illustrations to:

WHO and UNICEF for IMNCI

Clinical Methods in Paediatrics by Dr Raza-ur-Rehman

Clinical Methods in Paediatrics Diagnosis by Balu H. Athreya, MD

Pocket Essentials of Paediatrics, series editors; Parveen Kumar and Michael Clark

All attempts have been made to acknowledge the sources of information, omission if any, is regretted.

Author

Sultan Mustafa

Professor and Head of Department, Paediatrics and Neonatology

Karachi Medical and Dental College and Abbasi Shaheed Hospital, Karachi

Convener, University of Karachi, Final year MBBS.

Examiner and Supervisor

1. MCPS and FCPS, College of Physicians and Surgeons of Pakistan
2. MD and DCH, University of Karachi

Chief Editor

1. Journal of 'Paediatrics International, Pakistan'
2. Journal of 'Paediatric Allergy and Asthma'
3. Journal 'NutriKare'
4. News bulletin 'Paediatric NEWS'

Author

1. 'Clinical Methods in Paediatrics'
2. 'Bedside Paediatrics'
3. 'Handbook of Paediatric Dosage'
4. 'Current Paediatric Protocol'
5. 'Paediatric BCQs and EMQs'

Reviewer

JCPSP, JPMA, IMJ and JPPA

Member, Faculty of Paediatrics, CPSP

President, Pakistan Paediatrics Association, Karachi Chapter (2012–14)

Inspector, Pakistan Medical and Dental Council, PMDC

Co-author

Dr Sumbal Waheed, MD

Senior Registrar, Department of Paediatrics, KMDC and ASH

Assistant Editor, Journal of 'Paediatrics International, Pakistan'

Assistant Editor, 'Paediatrics News'

Facilitator, IMNCI Workshops

Co-author

1. Current Paediatric Protocol
2. Paediatric BCQs and EMQs

History Taking

- Presenting Complaints
- History of Presenting Complaints
- Specific Points in History
- Past History
- Drug History
- Family History
- Birth History
- Vaccination History
- Developmental History
- Nutritional History
- Socio-economic History
- System Review
- Common Paediatric Symptoms
- Common Paediatric Signs

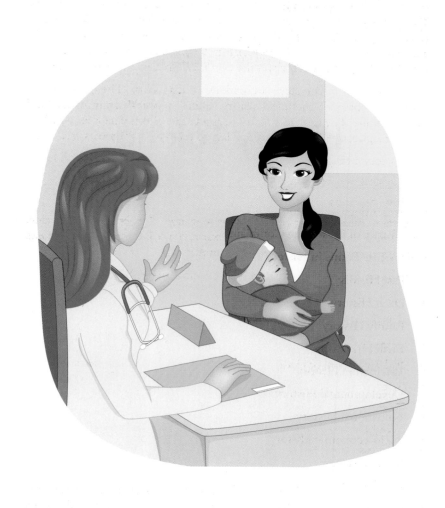

History Taking

A good history is more informative than examination and investigations. The history should be received, not extracted. Do not wear a white laboratory coat. Shake hands with both parents and child with a smile. The essential preliminary to any history taking is the establishment of eye contact between the doctor and the patient. Don't get the gender wrong.

There are two main steps in making a diagnosis. The first step is clinical database, it includes history taking, physical examination and investigations. The second step is interpretation of this database to make a proper diagnosis. The three basic pillars to establish a diagnosis are:

- History taking
- Physical examination
- Investigations

In certain cases examination will be negative. e.g. epilepsy, migraine. The reverse may also be true when examination is more conclusive e.g. leukaemia, nephrotic syndrome, pneumonia etc.

Note down the preliminary data before taking proper history.

Preliminary Data

- Name
- Age (with date of birth)
- Sex
- Race
- Weight
- Address
- Date of admission

Gender is important in diseases related to sex organs and genetically determined disorders. Some X linked disorders are common in males e.g. haemophilia. Age is also important from the point of view of incidence, severity and prognosis of diseases and dosage of drugs to be prescribed. The different paediatric age groups are described in table 1.1. Race is important because some diseases are more common in certain ethnic communities. Residence is important specially when a disease is epidemic or endemic in that area.

Table 1.1   Paediatric age groups

Neonate	Birth to 28 days
Infant	Birth to 1 year
Toddler	1 year–3 years
Pre-school age	3 years–5 years
School going age	5 years–15 years

Presenting Complaints

Record the immediate important complaints, which have led the parents to seek medical advice. They should be recorded in a chronological order i.e symptoms of longer duration come first. For example,

- Fever for five days

- Abdominal pain for three days

- Vomiting since morning

History of Presenting Complaints

A useful opening question is 'when was the child last feeling well?'. Allow parents to tell the story in their own words. Listen carefully and observe the child at this stage: activity, cry, expression, awareness and responsiveness. It is important to remember that many parents need assistance and guidance to avoid going off the track. The parents and the child should preferably be given a choice in many directions so that information is objective. In general, the following points should be noted:

Onset of Symptoms

- Acute (e.g. bronchial asthma, pneumothorax)

- Subacute (e.g. pneumonia, measles)

- Insidious (e.g. tuberculosis, typhoid)

Progress of Symptoms

- Improving (e.g. migraine, epilepsy)
- Waxing and waning (e.g. nephrotic syndrome, rheumatism)
- Progressive (e.g. leukaemia, degenerative disease)

Associated Symptoms

Example: Fever with abdominal pain and headache is seen in enteric fever, fever with weight loss and cough is a feature of tuberculosis or sore throat and abdominal pain may be a feature of tonsillitis.

Aggravating or Relieving Factors

Example: Cough is sometimes aggravated by dust or smoke. It is sometimes relieved by using bronchodilators as seen in asthma.

Medical Treatment

Mention any medications received during the illness. Mention the name of drugs, dosage and duration of treatment.

Negative Data

Persistant negative data should be obtained by direct questions. Some paediatricians prefer to obtain a systemic review.

SPECIFIC POINTS IN HISTORY

Note the following points in relation to specific symptoms:

Blood in Stool

- How often
- Colour
- Only blood or mixed with mucous

- Pain before blood
- Constipation
- Abdominal pain during defaecation
- Any other bleeding site

Constipation

- Onset
- Dietary relation (feeding habits, fluid intake, fibre)
- Any other abdominal symptoms like pain or vomiting.
- Any loss of weight
- Change in family life

Convulsions

- First or recurrent
- Febrile or afebrile
- Any systemic illness like cardiac, hepatic or renal disease.
- History of trauma
- History of drug intake
- Birth history

Cough

- Duration
- Severity
- Dry or productive
- Colour of sputum
- Associated fever
- Any chest pain
- Character of cough (e.g. whooping, aphonic, hoarse cough etc.)
- Daytime or nighttime, bouts or episodic.

Crying

- Loud
- High-pitched
- Stridorous
- Feeble
- Continuous
- Intermittent
- Grunting cry
- Cat like cry
- Masculine cry
- Cry on handling

Diarrhoea

- Duration
- Severity
- Volume
- Colour
- Is there any vomiting?
- Any abdominal pain
- Is there any blood or mucous?
- Urine output
- Any weight loss
- Is the child thirsty or drinks eagerly?

Dyspnoea

- Any fever
- Any cough
- Recurrent

- At rest or on exertion
- Any cyanosis
- Abnormally sleepy or difficult to wake
- Is the child taking orally?
- Breathing fast or normally

Oedema

- Generalised or localised
- Symmetrical or asymmetrical
- Associated abdominal distention
- Any scrotal swelling
- Nutritional intake
- Any dyspnoea or cyanosis
- Any history of jaundice
- Urinary output

Enuresis

- During day or night
- Child ever had bladder control
- Family history
- Urine volume
- Recent stress

Fever

- Onset and duration of fever
- Continuous, intermittent or remittent
- Associated chills
- Any episode of convulsion

- High grade or low grade
- Any focal symptoms

Headache

- Frontal, temporal or occipital
- Duration
- Severity
- Worse in morning or end of the day
- Associated vomiting
- Any visual symptoms
- Colour of urine

Jaundice

- Age of onset
- Colour of stool
- Colour of urine
- Any itching
- Abdominal symptoms
- Any drug history
- History of blood transfusion

Joint Pain

- Onset (Acute or insidious)
- History of trauma
- Single or multiple joint involvement
- Migratory or non-migratory
- Is there any rash?
- Any gastrointestinal, eye or bleeding disorder

Rash

- Generalised or localised
- Symmetrical or asymmetrical
- Type of rash
- Any prodromal phase
- Relation with prodrome
- Distribution of rashes
- Progression
- Duration
- Associated itching

Vomiting

- Age of onset
- Associated diarrhoea
- History of weight loss
- Systemic symptoms
- Is it projectile?
- Relation with feeding
- Material in vomitus
- Drug history

Pain

- Location
- Severity
- Duration
- What brings it about
- Does anything relieves it
- Periodicity
- Associated symptoms
- Timing
- Characteristics

Past History

Details of all minor and major diseases are required. Details of past accident, previous infections (e.g. tuberculosis, pneumonia, gastroenteritis, measles etc), ingestion of toxin, history of operations, history of similar illness (e.g. nephrotic syndrome, acute rheumatic fever etc), blood transfusion and hospital admission are to be included in this section.

Drug History

Any regular medication like bronchodilator, steroid etc. Any untoward side effects with any drugs.

Family History

This includes history of siblings and history of parents. The number, age and sex of siblings. Did any sibling die because of any known or unknown cause. Detail regarding age, health and any disease affecting parents are also required. Consanguinity between parents is important for genetic disorders.

Birth History

It is divided into three headings:

1. Antenatal
2. Natal
3. Post natal

Antenatal History

Enquire about:

*   Nutritional status of mother
*   Maternal intake of iron, multivitamin or drugs
*   Maternal illness during pregnancy
*   Exposure to radiation
*   Any problems with previous pregnancies like abortion, stillbirth etc.

Natal History

Enquire about:

- Place of delivery (hospital, clinic, home)
- Person who conducted the delivery (trained or untrained e.g. dai)
- Duration of pregnancy
- Mode of delivery (NVD, LSCS, forceps)
- Duration of labour
- Any drug used during labour

Post Natal History

Enquire about:

- Apgar score
- Birth weight
- Did the child cry immediately
- Was child cyanosed or apneic?
- Any history of post natal illness
- Any history of jaundice, phototherapy, exchange transfusion or umblical catheterisation,
- Any medication during neonatal period.

Vaccination History

Enquire about the age, at which the vaccination was started, number of doses received, any reaction to vaccination and enquire about the booster dose (for details, see chapter of vaccination).

Developmental History

There are several long and detailed volumes written about childhood development. One needs details of the milestones, if a child is brought for developmental delay. Beware of the great variation in developmental achievement. It may be normal for a child to walk precociously at 10 months. It is critical that the paediatrician can detect the subtle abnormalities and normal variation so that he or she can explain confidently to the anxious parents.

The developmental aspect of child is divided into four broad categories:

1. Gross motor
2. Fine motor
3. Social
4. Language

Denver's developmental screening chart is very useful for assessing the development of a child. However, the rapid summary here, will give the paediatrician a reliable guide to the developmental milestones most commonly seen. (see chapter of developmental screening). See table 1.2 for rapid bedside screening.

Table 1.2   Rapid bedside developmental screening

Milestones	Age
• Social smile	1 month
• Neck holding	3 months
• Supported sit	6 months
• Unsupported sit/transfer object from one hand to other hand	7 months
• Hold object between thumb and fingers	8 months
• Supported stand	9 months
• Walk with support	10 months
• Unsupported stand	11 months
• Attempt to walk alone	12 months
• Run	18 months
• Sphincter control	24 months
• Speech (1–2 words)	12 months

Nutritional History

Was the baby breastfed or bottle fed?

If the baby is breastfed then enquire about the following:

- Duration of exclusive breastfeeding
- How often did she feed?
- Does the baby sleep after feeding?
- On demand feeding or some feeding schedule
- Is the baby gaining weight?

If the baby is bottle fed then enquire about the following:

- Reason for bottle feeding
- Age at which the bottle was started.
- Dilution technique
- Amount of milk per feed
- Frequency of feeding
- Sterilisation technique
- Other fluids

When was weaning started and enquire about the following:

- Type of weaning
- Likes or dislikes
- Problems during weaning
- Is the child gaining weight?
- Any food allergies
- Amount of calories and protein contents in the diet
- Any multivitamins or iron supplementation

Socio-economic History

Enquire about occupation and income of the parents, living arrangements whether it is an extended family, nuclear family or a single parent family and what are the sources of support for the mother in physical, emotional and financial areas. Details of the house particularly about number and size of rooms, ventilation, sewerage system, availability of clean water and hygienic conditions of the surroundings are also important in assessing the socio-economic status of the family.

> 'A committee is a group of people who individually can do nothing but together can decide that nothing can be done.'
>
> **Fred Allen**

History Taking-Summary

Preliminary data

- Name
- Age
- Sex
- Race
- Weight
- Address
- Date of admission

Presenting complaints

History of presenting complaints

- Onset of symptoms
- Progress of symptoms
- Associated symptoms
- Aggravating or relieving factors
- Medical treatment received
- Persistent negative data

Past history

Drug history

Family history

Birth history

- Antenatal
- Natal
- Postnatal

Vaccination history

Developmental history

Nutritional history

Socio-economic status

System Review

There is no need to repeat previously recorded information in writing a review of systems.

- **General:** Unusual weight gain or loss, fatigue, temperature sensitivity, mentality. Pattern of growth (record previous heights and weights on appropriate graphs). Time and pattern of pubescence.

- **Skin:** Ask about rashes, hives, problems with hair, skin texture or colour, etc.

- **Eyes:** Have the child's eyes ever been crossed? Any foreign body or infection, glasses for any reason.

- **Ears, Nose and Throat:** Frequent colds, sore throat, sneezing, stuffy nose, discharge, post-nasal drip, mouth breathing, snoring, otitis, hearing, and adenitis.

- **Teeth:** Age of eruption of deciduous and permanent; number at one year; comparison with siblings.

- **Cardio respiratory:** Frequency and nature of disturbances. Dyspnea, chest pain, cough, sputum, wheeze, expectoration, cyanosis, oedema, syncope, tachycardia.

- **Gastrointestinal:** Vomiting, diarrhoea, constipation, type of stools, abdominal pain or discomfort, jaundice.

- **Genitourinary:** Enuresis, dysuria, frequency, polyuria, pyuria, haematuria, character of stream, vaginal discharge, menstrual history, bladder control, abnormalities of penis or testes.

- **Neuromuscular:** Headache, nervousness, dizziness, tingling, convulsions, habit spasms, ataxia, muscle or joint pains, postural deformities, exercise tolerance, gait.

- **Endocrine:** Disturbances of growth, excessive fluid intake, polyphagia, goiter, thyroid disease.

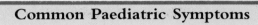

Common Paediatric Symptoms

Common Complaints	Common Diagnoses	Significant Other Diagnoses to Consider
Cough	URTI Pneumonia Croup Bronchiolitis Bronchitis Asthma Sinusitis	Cystic fibrosis Pertussis Tuberculosis Foreign body aspiration GE reflux Chlamydia pneumonitis
Fever	Viral fever Malaria Enteric fever Dengue fever Occult bacteremia UTI, pyelonephritis Viral exanthems Scarlet fever	Osteomyelitis Meningitis Febrile convulsions Septic arthritis Kawasaki's disease JRA Viral exanthem Tuberculosis
Sore throat	Pharngitis Scarlet fever Tonsillitis Cervical adenitis Pharyngeal and retropharyngeal abscesses	Rheumatic fever
Earache	Otitis media Otitis externa	Foreign body Mastoiditis
URTI	Conjunctivitis Allergic rhinitis Sinusitis Pharngitis	

Abdominal pain	Appendicitis	Intussusception
	UTI/Pyelonephritis	HS Purpura
	Gastroenteritis	Inflammatory bowel disease
	Constipation	Ulcer
	PID	Ovarian/testicular torsion
	Gastritis	Abdominal mass/malignancy
	Colic	Wilm's tumour
	Hepatitis	Neuroblastoma
	Encopresis	Lymphoma
	Psychogenic abdominal pain	Hydronephrosis
		Hernia
Vomiting	GE reflux	Volvulus/bowel obstruction
	Pyloric stenosis	Diabetic ketoacidosis
	Gastroenteritis	Increase intracranial pressure
	2nd to infections-	Hepatitis
	Pharngitis	Pyelonephritis
	Otitis media	
	Pneumonia	
	Meningitis	
Diarrhoea +/-vomiting	Gastroenteritis	Malnutrition
	Giardiasis	Haemolytic uremic syndrome
	Dysentery	Malobsorbtion syndrome
	Parental	
Skin problems	Urticaria	Anaphylaxis
	Atopic dermatitis	Drug reaction rash
	Contact dermatitis	Stevens Johnson syndrome
	Fungal infections	Seborrheic dermatitis
	Scabies	
	Impetigo/cellulitis	
	Tinea infections	

Limp/limb pain	Trauma	Arthritis (JRA)
	Tendonitis Toxic synovitis Infectious –	Sickle cell crisis
	Septic arthritis	Rheumatic fever
	Osteomyelitis	Leukaemia/tumours
	Cellulitis	
Headache	Migraine	Increased intracranial pressure
	Tension	Increased blood pressure
	Meningitis	
	URTI	
	Visual problem	

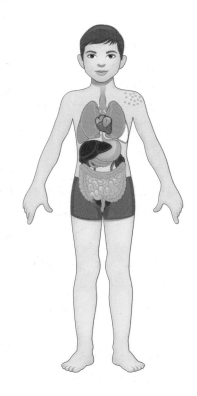

Common Paediatric Signs

Common Signs	Common Diseases	Significant Other Diagnoses to Consider
Heart murmur	Innocent murmurs Cardiac defects	Acute rheumatic fever Congestive cardiac failure
Lymphadenopathy	Infectious mononucleosis Bacterial adenitis Viral infections Systemic infections e.g. Tuberculosis	Kawasaki's disease lymphoma/ leukaemia HIV/ AIDS Cat scratch disease
Splenomegaly	Systemic infectious disease e.g. Malaria, Enteric fever etc Haemolytic anaemias	Tumours Sickle cell disease
Hepatomegaly	Hepatitis Systemic infectious disease e.g. Malaria, Enteric fever etc	Congestive heart failure Cirrhosis
Impaired vision	Strabismus/amblyopia Myopia/hyperopia Leucocoria	Retinoblastoma Cataracts
Pallor/anaemia	Iron deficiency anaemia Thalassaemia Lead poisoning Occult blood loss	Haemolytic anaemias Malignancy

Bruising/ Petechiae	HS Purpura Leukaemia Secondary to infection Trauma Vasculitis ITP	Haemophilia/Von Willebrand's
Haematuria	Acute Glomerulonephritis Trauma UTI Haemolytic uremic syndrome HS Purpura SLE	IgA Nephropathy
Proteinuria	Nephrotic syndrome Acute Glomerulonephritis Orthostatic Proteinuria	Metabolic renal disease

CHAPTER 02

General Examination

- Signs of Acute Illness
- General Appearance
- State of Nutrition
- Face and Facial Expressions
- Cry or Voice
- Skin
- Hands
- Neck
- Two Routines
- Vital Signs
- Physical Parameters
- Weight
- Height
- Occipito-Frontal Circumference (OFC)
- Examination Review-Check List

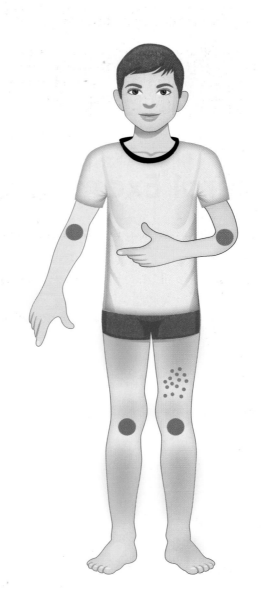

General Examination

It is essential to develop a confident ease, which transmits itself to the parents and most important of all to the child. Once a symptom becomes familiar, the maximum information can be obtained gently and efficiently with the minimum of upset. The following preliminary guidelines should be kept in mind before examining a child:

- Avoid having children separated from parents, forcibly undressed and measured, if possible
- Give infant something to hold
- The room and hands should be warm. Keep small number of people in the room.
- Continue to talk quietly and gently throughout the examination
- Collect all information available in any sequence
- When the child is asleep, then it is better to auscultate chest, palpate abdomen and do fundoscopy first

Following are the possible sequence of collecting information:

1. Assess signs of acute illness
2. General appearance
3. State of nutrition
4. Facial expression
5. Cry or voice
6. Skin
7. Hands
8. Neck
9. Two routines
10. Vital signs
11. Physical parameters.

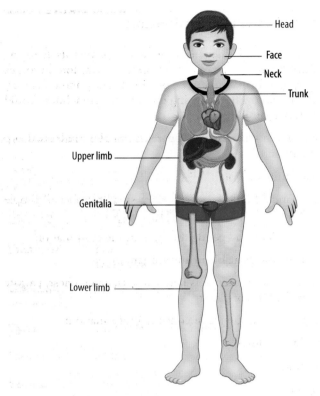

Fig. 2.1 Head to Toe examination.

1. Signs of Acute Illness

The first step is to ascertain whether the child is well, mildly ill or severely ill. Presence of any of the signs in the following list should indicate a serious problem and require immediate attention:

- Haemorrhagic rash
- Cyanosis
- Grunting
- Gasping or apnea
- Respiratory distress
- Decreased activity or Flaccidity

- Abnormal posture

- Dehydration

- Distended abdomen

- Stridor or wheezing

- Convulsions or drowsiness

These can be detected by a rapid look as skin, cry, respiration, activity, posture, eyes and abdomen.

IMCI (Integrated Management of Childhood Illnesses) describes triage of all sick children which divides the severity of illness into three groups on the basis of signs present in the child. These are emergency signs, priority signs and non-urgent signs (see table 2.1). Children with emergency signs require immediate treatment. The priority signs identify children who are at a higher risk of dying. These children should be assessed without delay.

Table 2.1   Assesment of severity of a child according to IMNCI

Emergency signs	Priority signs
Airway and breathing	• Visible severe wasting
• Obstructed breathing	• Oedema of both feet
• Central cyanosis	• Severe palmer pallor
• Severe resp. distress	• Sick infant less than two months
Circulation	• Lethargic or drowsy
• Cold hands (sign of circulatory failure)	• Irritable or restless
	• Any respiratory distress
Coma or convulsion	• Major burns
Severe dehydration	

2. General Appearance

Is the child looking ill, toxic, drowsy, lethargic, active, responsive, aware, irritable, stuporous or comatose? Signs of acute illness are mentioned in general appearance.

3. State of Nutrition

One has to know whether the child is overweight, lean, marasmic or dehydrated (see table 2.2). The differentiating point between marasmus and kwashiorkor are described in table 2.3.

4. Face and Facial Expressions

Face is the index of mind and mirror of many diseases. It may be toxic, dehydrated, marasmic, pale, mongoloid, cretin, tetanic, thalassemic, cushingoid or dysmorphic. It is also diagnostic in facial nerve palsy, ocular nerve palsy and measles.

Table 2.2   Assessment of dehydration

Features	No Dehydration	Some Dehydration	Severe Dehydration
General appearance	Normal	Lethargic	Drowsy or unconscious
Eyes	Normal	Sunken	Sunken and dry
Mouth	Moist	Dry	Very dry
Fontanelle	Normal	Depressed	Very Depressed
Skin turgor	Normal	Goes back slowly < 2 second	Goes back slowly > 2 second
Pulse	Normal	Weak and rapid	Impalpable

5. Cry or Voice

Some of the causes associated with peculiar cry are listed below:

Loud Lusty Cry

- Full term newborn
- Healthy child
- Hunger

- Wet child

- Change in temperature

- Temper tantrum

Feeble Cry

- Acute illness

- Severe tantrum

- Beri beri

- Down syndrome

Table 2.3   Features of nutritional syndromes

Marasmus	Kwashiorkor
1. The child is lethargic or irritable	1. The child looks apathetic
	2. Oedema, pitting in nature
2. Loose skin folds due to the loss of subcutaneous fat	3. Hair changes: (dry, coarse, depigmented, loss of curliness and plucked out painlessly)
3. Old man look due to the loss of buccal pad of fat	
4. Severe muscle wasting	4. Skin changes: (hyperpigmentation, depigmentation, desquamation, wet-oozing skin and haemorrhage)
5. Prominent rib cage	
	5. Enlarged liver due to fatty infiltration

High-Pitched Cry

- Intracranial lesion

- Kernicterus

- Hydrocephalus

Continuous Cry

Mental retardation

Intermittent Cry

- Colic
- Intussusception

Cat Cry

- Cri-du-chat syndrome
- Masculine cry
- Precocious puberty

Grunting Cry

- Pneumonia
- Emphysema

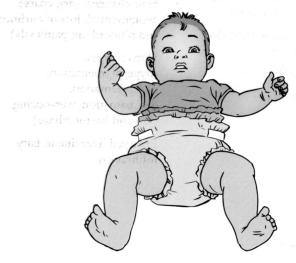

Fig. 2.2   Asymmetrical tonic neck reflex.

Hoarse Cry

- Cretinism
- Laryngitis
- Diphtheria

6. Skin

Before inspecting any rash, note the colour of the skin. It may be pale, abnormally red, flushed, cyanosis or jaundice. Also note the area of altered pigmentation. Methods of eliciting anaemia, jaundice, cyanosis and oedema are summarised in table 2.5, 2.6, 2.7 and 2.8.

Haemorrhage in the skin is very important to detect. It may be purpura, ecchymosis or haematoma. Whenever you detect any skin lesion (table 2.4), following points should be noted:

- Symmetrical or asymmetrical
- Centrifugal or centripetal
- Flexor or extensor bias
- Localised or generalised
- Irritation

Table 2.4   Types of skin lesions

Macule	Area of discolouration, not raised, depressed or thickened
Papule	Palpable elevation of the skin up to 5 mm in diameter;
Nodule	Larger than papules, may be soft, hard, cutaneous or subcutaneous.
Vesicle	Blister of up to 5 mm diameter filled with serous fluid (if opaque and yellow then called pustule)
Bullae	Larger blister
Weals	Oedematous elevation of the skin
Fissures	Small cracks in the epidermis, exposing the dermis
Ulcer	Destruction of whole thickness of the skin
Lichenification	Thickened skin due to the chronic irritation

Table 2.5   Anaemia

Definition:	Decrease haemoglobin or red blood cells per unit volume of blood
Site for looking:	Nails, lower conjunctiva, hard palate, palmer crease
Common causes:	Haemolytic, haemorrhagic, nutritional, bone marrow failure

Table 2.6   Cyanosis

Definition:	Blue discolouration of skin and mucous membrane.
Type:	Peripheral and central
Site for looking:	Nails (peripheral), lips (central)
Causes of Central cyanosis:	Cyanotic congenital heart disease, pulmonary disease, eisenmenger syndrome.
Causes of Peripheral cyanosis:	Shock, congestive cardiac failure, exposure to cold

Table 2.7   Jaundice

Definition:	Yellow discolouration of skin and mucous membrane due to increased bilirubin in body fluids.
Site for looking:	Sclera, mucous membrane of mouth, skin
Common causes:	Haemolytic anaemia, hepatitis, cholestasis

Table 2.8   Oedema

Definition:	Excessive accumulation of extravascular fluid
Site for looking:	Medial malleoli, Sacrum, Periorbital
Common causes:	Cardiac failure, nephrotic syndrome, kwashiorkor, hepatic failure, protein losing enteropathy

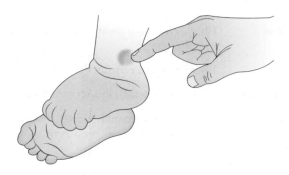

Fig. 2.3   Method of checking ankle oedema:

7. Hands

Look for pallor, jaundice, cyanosis, clubbing, koilonychia, splinter haemorrhage, swelling (soft tissue or bony) and any obvious deformity either congenital or acquired.

In true clubbing, the height at the base of the nails is greater than at the distal interphalangeal joints. Clubbing may be idiopathic, familial or because of long standing systemic disease (cardiac, pulmonary, gastrointestinal and hepatic). See table 2.14. Splinter haemorrhage are small subungual linear haemorrhage, caused by trauma, subacute bacterial endocarditis, blood dyscrasias, sickle cell anaemia, infectious mononucleosis.

Koilonychia is soft brittle and spoon shape nail, may be because of iron deficiency, protein malnutrition, familial or idiopathic.

8. Neck

Examine lymph nodes (see table 2.9), thyroid gland, submandibular salivary gland, parotid gland, carotid pulse and venous pulse(see chapter on examination of cardiovascular system).

9. Two Routines

Test for congenital dislocation of hip joint and radio-femoral pulse delay should be checked on all newborns and infants routinely.

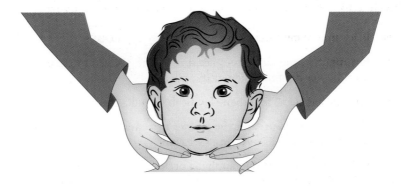

Fig. 2.4   Method of palpating cervical lymph nodes:

Table 2.9   Lymph node examination

Sites for looking:	Suboccipital, retro-auricular, parotid, sub mandibular, submental, superficial cervical, supraclavicular, axillary, inguinal and epitrochlear
Note the following:	Location, tenderness, mobility, adherence matting, overlying skin and consistency
Common causes of enlarged lymph node:	Infection, tuberculosis, lymphoma, leukaemia, infectious mononucleosis, kawasaki disease etc.

Congenital Dislocation of Hip Joint

Following are the signs of congenital hip dislocation:

1.   Asymmetrical gluteal and thigh folds

2.   Barlow modification of Ortolanis maneuver. (table 2.10)

3.   Allis sign: When hips and knees are flexed, the knees are at unequal heights with dislocation side lower

4.   Trendlenberg gait

Table 2.10   Barlows modification of Ortolani's maneuver:

- Place the infant on its back.

- Examiner's long finger is placed over the greater trochanter and thumb over the inner side of the thigh.

- Hips flexed at 90° and then slowly abducted.

- With gentle pressure, lift the greater trochanter forward, a slipping sensation is felt (dislocation)-Ortolani.

- If the joint is more stable, applying of slight pressure with the thumb, as the thigh is abducted, slipping the hip posteriorly (dislocatable)-Barlow's modification.

Radio-Femoral Delay

Femoral pulse is felt at a point midway between the symphysis pubis and anterior superior iliac spine. One should feel the radial artery while feeling the femoral artery. In the presence of coarctation of aorta, there is delay between femoral and radial pulse and difference in the volume of the pulse will be present.

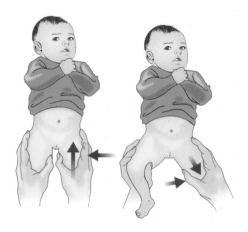

Fig. 2.5   Examination of Hip Joint.

10. Vital Signs

Temperature

It can be recorded by different routes: oral, axillary or rectal. The last method is preferred in neonates and infancy.

Rectal temperature is 1 degree F higher than oral temperature and axillary temperature is 1 degree F lower than oral temperature. There are three classical patterns of fever:

1. **Continuous:** Daily fluctuations do not exceed 1 degree C.

2. **Remittent:** Daily fluctuations exceed 2 degree C but never touch the normal.

3. **Intermittent:** Temperature touches normal for several hours in a day.

Pulse

The radial, brachial, carotid, femoral, popliteal, posterior tibial and dorsalis pedis should be noted. Radial pulse is felt with the tips of the fingers against the head of the radius while forearm is slightly pronated and wrist slightly flexed. Following observations should be noted:

1. Rate

2. Rhythm

3. Volume

4. Character

5. Comparison of both sides

6. Radiofemoral delay

To assess the rate and rhythm, radial pulse is generally used. For volume and character one should examine the carotid artery. Normal pulse rates at different age groups are described in table 2.11.

Table 2.11   Pulse rates at different ages:

Age	Rate/minute (Ranges)
Newborn	70–170
Up to 1 year	80–160
2 years	80–130
4 years	80–120
6 years	75–115
8–10 years	70–110
Adolescent	65–110
Adult	60–100

Blood Pressure (Table 2.12)

Blood pressure measurement is often a neglected portion of the physical examination of children. There are different types of instruments used to measure blood pressure but the mercury and aneroid type of sphygmomanometers are the commonly used instrument in clinical practise. For children, select the cuff size which covers most of the upper arm but leaves a gap of 1 cm below the axilla and above the antecubital fossa. A narrow cuff will give a high reading and a broader cough will give a lower blood pressure. In suspected coarctation of aorta it may be useful to compare the systolic blood pressure in arm with that in the leg. Use 18 cm cuff, applied above the knee, with patient facing downward and auscultate over popliteal artery.

Table 2.12   Method of measuring blood pressure:

- Apply deflated appropriate size cuff over upper arm in sitting or lying position.
- Inflate cuff, 10–20 mm high above the point at which the pulsation of radial artery disappears.
- Palpate brachial artery and place the stethoscope over it.
- Deflate cuff pressure, 2–3 mm Hg/beat.
- The point, at which first heart sound is heard, is the systolic pressure
- Continue to deflate, the sound suddenly becomes faint or muffled and disappear.
- Diastolic pressure is best measured at the point of complete disappearance of the sound.
- Plot the reading on a centile chart and decide accordingly.

Respiratory Rate

Note the respiratory rate for one minute when at rest or while sleeping. Other characteristics are also noted: rhythm, depth, adventitious sound, odour of breathing and signs of respiratory distress. The cut off point of tachypnea for different age groups are as follows:

- 0–2 months >60 breaths/min
- 2–12 months >50 breaths/min
- 1–5 years >40 breaths/min
- After 5 years > 30 breaths/min

11. Physical Parameters

It includes the following:

- Weight
- Height
- Occipitofrontal Circumference (OFC)
- Mid Arm Circumference (MAC)
- Mid Chest Circumference (MCC)

- Body proportions
- Dentitions
- Ossification centers

The most important being weight, height and OFC, they will be described here in detail.

Weight

It should be done routinely for all children especially < 3 years and those having risk factors for malnutrition. Preferably taken on the same machine with minimal clothing. The scale should be checked for accuracy by using standard weights. There are different methods for assessing weight gain pattern but the most reliable way is by using standard formulas:

- 3–12 months: (Age in month +9)/2   = Weight (kg)
- 6 year: Age (years) x 2 + 8   = Weight (kg)
- 7–12 year: (Age in years x 7–5)/2   = Weight (kg)

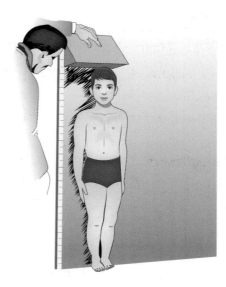

Fig. 2.6   Method of measuring height.

Height

In infants and children below 2–3 years, it should be measured in a lying position (length) while in older children in standing position (stature). During measurement, make sure that feet are held together, back straight and eyes looking straight. The birth length is 50 cms, it increases by 2 cms/month, at 1 year it is 75 cms. After 2 years it is calculated by formula, up to the age of 12 years.

Height (cms) = Age (year) x 6 +77

Occipitofrontal Circumference (OFC)

It reflects the brain growth. It should be measured with a non-stretchable tape at the maximum point of occipital protuberance posteriorly and above the eyebrows anteriorly. It is 35 cms at birth and increases by 1 cm/month, it is 47 cms up to one year of age, it is also calculated by using the formula:

$$\frac{\text{Length (cms)} + 9.5 \pm 2.5}{2}$$

Up to one year it is 60% of the adult and at two year it is 75% of the adult size(see table 2.13).

Table 2.13   Occipitofrontal circumference at different ages

Age	OFC
Birth	35 cms
3 months	41 cms
6 months	44 cms
9 months	46 cms
1 year	47 cms
2 years	49 cms
3 years	50 cms
3–12 years	0.5 cm/year
	max. up to 54–56 cms

Table 2.14 Diseases associated with acquired digital clubbing:

Cardiac	Gastrointestinal
• Cyanotic congenital heart disease	• Coeliac disease
• Subacute bacterial endocarditis	• Chronic dysentery
	• Ulcerative colitis
	• Regional enteritis
Pulmonary	
• Abscess	**Hepatic**
• Bronchiectasis	• Biliary cirrhosis
• Chronic pneumonia	• Chronic active hepatitis
• Cystic fibrosis	
• Empyema	**Other**
• Tuberculosis	• Hodgkin disease
	• Thyrotoxicosis

General Examination-Summary:

1. Assess sign of acute illness
2. General appearance
3. State of nutrition
4. State of hydration
5. Facial expression
6. Cry or voice
7. Skin
   ○ Oedema
   ○ Anaemia
   ○ Cyanosis
   ○ Jaundice
   ○ Haemorrhage
8. Hands
9. Neck
   ○ Lymph nodes
   ○ Salivary glands
   ○ Venous pulse
   ○ Thyroid gland
10. Two Routines
    ○ Radio-femoral delay
    ○ Hip joint dislocation
11. Vital Sign
    ○ Pulse
    ○ Respiratory rate
    ○ Blood pressure
    ○ Temperature
12. Physical parameter
    ○ Weight
    ○ Height
    ○ Occipito-frontal circumference
    ○ Mid-arm circumference
    ○ Mid-chest circumference
    ○ Dentition
    ○ Body proportion
    ○ Arm span

Examination Review-Checklist

1. General Appearance

- Does the child appear well or ill?
- State of hydration, nutrition and circulation
- Consciousness, gait, posture, and coordination
- Nature of cry and degree of activity,
- Facies and facial expression

2. Vital Signs

- Temperature
- Pulse rate, and
- Respiratory rate (TPR);
- Blood pressure (the cuff should cover 2/3 of the upper arm)

3. Parameters

- Weight,
- Height, and
- Head circumference

4. Head

- Size and shape
- Circumference, asymmetry
- Cephalhaematoma or caput
- Frontal bossing and craniotabes
- Fontanel (size, tension, number, abnormally late or early closure), Sutures
- Dilated veins

- Scalp, hair (texture distribution)
- Transillumination

5. Face

- Dysmorphic facial features
- Sign of facial nerve palsy
- Tenderness over sinuses
- Parotid swelling
- Sinus tenderness

6. Eyes

- Photophobia, visual acuity, muscular control, nystagmus
- Mongolian slant, brushfield spots, epicanthic folds
- Lacrimation, discharge, redness
- Exophthalmos or enophthalmos
- Pupillary size, shape, reaction to light and accommodation
- Corneal opacities, cataracts
- Fundi, visual fields (in older children)
- Signs of vitamin A deficiency

7. Nose

- Shape, mucosa, patency, discharge or bleeding
- Pressure over sinuses.
- Flaring of nostrils.

8. Mouth

- Lips (thinness, down turning, fissures, colour, cleft)
- Teeth (number, position, caries, mottling, discolouration. notching, malocclusion or mal alignment)

- Mucosa (colour, redness of Stensen's duct, enanthems, Bohn's nodules, Epstein's pearls).
- Gum, palate, tongue, uvula, mouth breathing, geographic tongue (usually normal).
- Sign of vitamin deficiencies(angular stomatitis,gelosis,gum bleeding)

9. Throat

- Tonsils (size, inflammation, exudates, crypts, inflammation of the anterior pillars).
- Mucosa, hypertrophic lymphoid tissue, postnasal drip, epiglottis
- Voice (hoarseness, stridor, grunting, type of cry, speech)
- The number and condition of the teeth should be recorded. (A child should have 20 teeth by age 2 years.

10. Ears

- Pinnas (position, size), canals
- Tympanic membranes (landmarks, mobility, perforation, inflammation, discharge). mastoid tenderness and swelling.
- Hearing screening

11. Neck

- Position (torticollis, opisthotonos, inability to support head, mobility). Thyroid (size, contour, bruit, isthmus, nodules, tenderness)
- Lymph nodes and JVP.
- Position of trachea.
- Sternocleidomastoid (swelling, shortening) or webbing of neck

12. Lymph Nodes

- Location, size, sensitivity, mobility, consistency and skin

- One should routinely attempt to palpate sub occipital, preauricular, anterior cervical, posterior cervical, sub maxillary, sublingual, axillary, epitrochlear, and inguinal lymph nodes.

13. Trunk

- Signs of PCM, rickets, skin turgor etc
- Check any other abnormalities like abdominal distension etc.

14. Hands

- Look for pallor, jaundice, cyanosis, clubbing, splinter haemorrhage and swelling.
- Any obvious deformity?

15. Foot

- Check oedema and pulsation in post.tibial artery.
- Any obvious deformity?

16. Skin

- Colour (cyanosis, jaundice, pallor, and erythema) and Pigmentation.
- Skin Lesio.
- Hydration, and Oedema
- Haemorrhagic manifestations.
- Hair distribution and character, and desquamation.

17. (a) Male Genitalia

- Circumcision, meatal opening, hypospadias, phimosis, adherent foreskin
- Size of testes, cryptorchidism
- Scrotum, hydrocele, hernia, pubertal changes

17. (b) Female Genitalia

- Vagina (imperforate, discharge, adhesions)
- Hypertrophy of clitoris
- Pubertal changes

18. Rectum and Anus

- Irritation, fissures, prolapse, imperforate anus.
- The rectal examination should be performed with the little finger (inserted slowly). Note muscle tone, character of stool, masses, tenderness, sensation.

System Review

Respiratory System

- Shape and symmetry, veins, retractions and pulsations, beading, Harrison's groove, flaring of ribs, pigeon breast, funnel shape, size and position of nipples, breasts, length of sternum, intercostals and substernal retraction.

- Type of breathing, dyspnea, prolongation of expiration and expansion.

- Fremitus, flatness or dullness to percussion.

- Resonance, breath and voice sounds, rales, wheezing

Cardiovascular System

- BP, JVP and pulses.

- Precordial bulging, pulsation of vessels, thrills, size, shape of precordium

- Auscultation (rate, rhythm, force, quality of sounds and intensity).

- Location and intensity of apex beat

- Murmurs (location, position in cycle, intensity, pitch, effect. of change of position, transmission and effect of exercise)

Abdomen

- Size and contour, visible peristalsis, respiratory movements, veins (distension, direction of flow), umbilicus, hernia, and scar mark.

- Tenderness, rebound tenderness and rigidity

- Fluid thrill and shifting dullness.

- Palpable organs or masses (size, shape, position, mobility)

- Bowel sounds

Neurologic Examination

- Cerebral function: general behaviour, level of consciousness, intelligence, emotional status, memory, orientation, recognition of visual object, speech, ability to write, performance of skilled motor acts

- Cranial nerves:

- Cerebellar Function: Finger to nose, finger to examiner's finger, rapidly alternating pronation and supination of hands; ability to run heel down other shin and to make a requested motion with foot; ability to stand with eyes closed; walk; heel to toe walk; tremor; ataxia; posture; arm swing when walking; nystagmus; abnormalities of muscle tone or speech

- Motor System: Muscle size, consistency, and tone; muscle contours and outlines; muscle strength; myotonic contraction; slow relaxation; symmetry or posture; fasciculations; tremor; resistance to passive movement; involuntary movement

- Sensory System: Hearing, vision, light touch, pain, position, vibration

- Deep reflexes: Biceps, brachioradialis, triceps, patellar, achilles and clonus. Superficial reflexes: Abdominals, cremasteric, plantar and gluteal

Musculoskeletal System

- General: Deformity, hemi hypertrophy, bowlegs (common in infancy), knock-knees (common after age 2), paralysis, oedema, coldness, posture, gait, stance, asymmetry.

- Joints: Swelling, redness, pain, limitation, tenderness, motion, rheumatic nodules, carrying angle of elbows, tibial torsion.

- Hands and feet: Extra digits, clubbing, simian lines, curvature of little finger, deformity of nails, splinter haemorrhages, flat feet (feet commonly appear flat during first 2 years), abnormalities of feet, dermatoglyphics, width of thumbs and big toes, syndactyly, length of various segments, dimpling of dorsa.

- Spine and Back-Posture, curvatures, rigidity, webbed neck, spina bifida, pilonidal dimple or cyst, tufts of hair, mobility, Mongolian spots, tenderness over spine, pelvis or kidneys.

CLASSIFICATION OF MALNUTRITION IN CHILDREN

Modified Gomez Classification

	Mild Malnutrition	Moderate Malnutrition	Severe Malnutrition
Percent Ideal body weight	71%-80%	61%-70%	<60%

Gomez Classification

Percent of reference weight for age	Interpretation
90–110%	Normal
75–89%	Grade I: mild malnutrition
60–74%	Grade II: moderate malnutrition
< 60%	Grade III: severe malnutrition

Wellcome Classification

Weight for age (Gomez)	With Oedema	Without Oedema
60–80%	Kwashiorkor	Under nutrition
< 60%	Marasmic-kwashiorkor	Marasmus

Waterlow Classification

Waterlow classification	Weight for height(wasting)	Height for age (stunting)
Normal	>90	>95
Mild	80–90	90–95
Moderate	70–80	85–90
Severe	< 70	< 85

CHAPTER 03

Developmental Screening

- Birth History
- Family History
- Milestones
- Examination

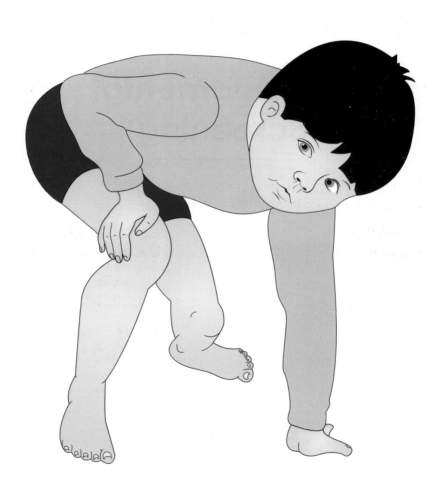

DEVELOPMENTAL SCREENING

Gesselle described sequence of development under four major categories:

- Gross motor
- Fine motor
- Language
- Personal–social

Many of the tests of child development in use today are modifications of Gessell's approach. The most popular of these tests is the Denver developmental screening test. It is not a diagnostic tool neither an intelligence test. Before assessing the child's development one should know the cause of developmental delay and normal ranges of development (Table 3.1, 3.2, 3.3) and take a detailed history.

Table 3.1   Causes of developmental delay

Types		Causes
Isolated delay	e.g.	Autism, cerebral palsy
Global delay	e.g.	Mental retardation
Neurological deficit	e.g.	Neurodegenerative disease
Structural deficit	e.g.	Congenital hip dislocation
Non organic	e.g.	Malnutrition, child abuse

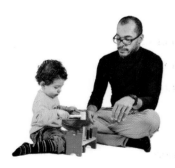

Fig. 3.1   Identifing colours and shapes

Table 3.2   Rapid bedside screening

Milestones	Age
• Smiling	1 month
• Neck holding	3 months
• Supported sit	6 months
• Unsupported sit/transfer object from one hand to other hand	7 months
• Holds object between thumb and fingers	8 months
• Supported stand	9 months
• Walk with support	10 months
• Unsupported stand	11 months
• Attempt to walk alone	12 months
• Run	18 months
• Sphincter control	24 months
• Speech (1–2 words)	12 months

Birth History

Birth history should include the following aspects:

Antenatal Factors

• Maternal illness

• Early ante-partum bleeding

• Maternal medication

• Exposure to radiation

Perinatal Factors

• Duration of gestation

• Duration of labour

- Duration of rupture of membrane
- Birth weight
- Abnormality of presentation
- APGAR score at 1, 5 and 20 minutes

Table 3.3   Normal ranges of development

Milestone	Range				
Smiling	Days		-	7	weeks
Sitting (with support)	5	months	-	1	year
Walking (with support)	8	months	-	4	years
Bladder control	15	months	-	10	years
Speech	10	months	-	5	years

Postnatal Factors
- Neonatal illness
- Neonatal jaundice
- Sucking or swallowing difficulties

Family History
- Family history of mental retardation or sub-normality
- Rate of development in family members
- Undue stress, emotional deprivation etc

Milestones
Note the following points:
- Isolated delay or global delay
- Milestones are slow, deteriorating or not developed

Examination

The physical examination must include the following:

- Physical parameters (weight, height, OFC)
- Congenital anomaly (dislocation of hip joint, meningomyelocele, etc)
- Signs of malnutrition
- Central nervous system (awareness, responsiveness, memory, intelligence, speech, cranial nerve, motor system, reflexes and sensory system).
- Sign of chronic illness (renal, hepatic, cardiac disease etc.)

The history and relevant examination should be interpreted cautiously to make a diagnosis, specially when the child is low birth weight and born before term.

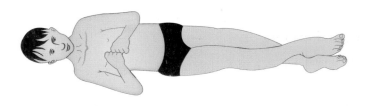

Fig. 3.2   Flexion of upper arm and scissoring of legs.

Newborn Examination

- Signs of acute illness
- Assessment of gestational age
- Recognition of congenital malformation
- Routine head to toe examination
- Primitive neonatal reflexes

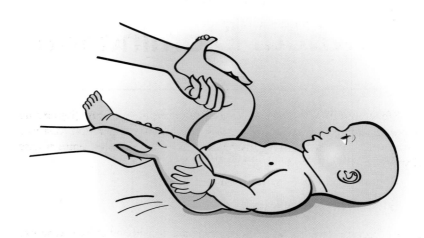

Newborn Examination

Every paediatrician must be able to recognise a sick newborn irrespective of his subspecialty and location of practise. It should be done as soon as convenient after birth. The objectives of examination are:

1. Assess signs of acute illness

2. Assessment of gestational age

3. Recognition of congenital malformation

4. Routine head to toe examination

5. Primitive neonatal reflexes

1. Signs of Acute Illness

Look for colour (pallor, cyanosis, jaundice and plethora), posture (hypotonic or opisthotonic), movement (jitteriness, convulsion), respiration (distress, retractions or grunting) responsiveness and other signs of acute illness (hypothermia, bleeding tendency etc).

2. Assessment of Maturity

Infants born before 37th week of gestation are considered to be premature and infants weighing 2.5 kg or less at birth are called Low Birth Weight (LBW). These infants are either preterm (< 37 weeks) or small for gestational age i.e. Intra uterine growth retardation.

There are various methods of assessing gestational age namely Parkin's criteria (table 4.1), Dubowtiz charting etc.

Since the development of the CNS correlates better with true gestational age than other criterion, it is better to use developmental reflexes to differentiate between premature infants and small for gestational age infant. For example:

- Sucking reflex   Absent < 31 weeks of GA

                   Present > 33 weeks of GA

- Rooting reflex   Absent < 31 weeks GA

                   Present > 33 weeks GA

- Moros reflex   Absent < 28 weeks GA

                           Present after 33 weeks GA

GA = Gestational Age.

Table 4.1   Parkin's criteria for assessing gestational age

	0	1	2	3	4
Skin texture	Thin and gelatinious	Thin and Smooth	Smooth and sup. peeling	Thick and stiff	Thick, parchment like
Skin colour	Deep red	Uniformly pink	Pale and pink	Pale except red ear, lips, palm and sole	
Breast size	Not palpable	Less than 0.5 cm	0.5–1 cm	Greater than 1 cm	
Ear firmness	Soft, easily folded and do not return	Soft, easily folded and slowly return	Cartilage felt at edge and rapidly return	Full cartilage at periphery and rapidly return	
Interpretation	Score-4 34.5 weeks	Score-5 36 weeks	Score-6 37 weeks	Score 11–12 42 weeks	+/-0–18 days, 95% confidence

3. Recognition of Congenital Malformations

These includes hydrocephalus, myelomeningocele, cleft lip, cleft palate, imperforate anus and congenital heart disease.

4. Routine Head to Toe Examination

It is best to proceed in a systemic fashion, starting from head and proceeding towards the toe. Also examine from back in a similar systemic way i.e. head to toe (see table 4.2)

5. Primitive Neonatal Reflexes

Important neonatal reflexes are described here. Absence or persistence of these reflexes beyond the period of which they should normally disappear indicates brain disorders.

Moros Reflex (Figure 4.1)

Method: Place infant supine, support the head with your hand, release the support, allowing the head to fall backwards for 10–15 cms on your other hand.

Response: Extension of arms, opening of hands followed by flexion and adduction of arms

Age of appearance (AA): 31st week of gestation Age of disappearance (AD): 3–4 months.

Startle Reflex

Method: Produce loud sound

Response: Similar to Moro

AA: Birth

AD: 3–4 months.

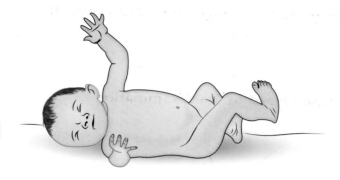

Fig. 4.1   Moro reflex in newborn.

Rooting Reflex

Method: Stroking the cheek

Response: Head turning towards stimulus

AA: 33 weeks of gestation

AD: Four months

Sucking Reflex

Method: Elevate head and introduce little finger into the mouth.

AA: 33 weeks of gestation

AD: Seven months

Placing Reflex

Method: Dorsal surface of one foot is drawn along the under surface of the table.

Response: Stimulated leg undergoes flexion

AA: Birth

AD: Six weeks

Palmer Grasp

Method: Place finger into the palm

Response: Closes the hand with firm grip

AA: Birth

AD: Six month

Glabellar Tap

Method: Sharp tap over glabella

Response: Momentary closure of eyes

AA: Birth

AD: Variable

Dolls Eye Reflex

Method: Turn head to one side

Response: Eye turn to opposite side

AA: Birth

AD: Two Weeks

Symmetrical Head Reflex

Method: Extension of head

Response: Extension of trunk and limbs

AA: Birth

AD: 8–10 weeks

Trunk in Curvature Reflex

Method: Stroke the paravertebral area.

Response: Lateral flexion of trunk

AA: Birth AD:

Three years.

Asymmetrical Tonic Neck Reflex (Figure 4.2)

Method: Turn the head of the supine infant rapidly to one side.

Response: Extension of the arms and legs on the side to which the head is turned and flexion of the arms and legs on the opposite side (fencing posture).

AA: Two months

AD: Six months

Stepping or Walking Reflex

Method: With the infant held upright and leaning forwards, the soles of the feet are allowed to touch the flat surface.

Response: Movement of progression.

AA: Birth

AD: Six weeks

Planter Grasp

Method: Press the finger over the distal part of the sole.

Response: Flexion of toes.

AA: Birth

AD: Ten months

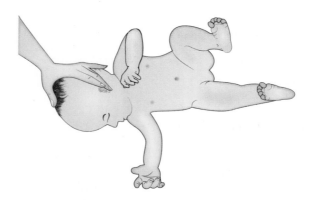

Fig. 4.2   Tonic neck reflex in newborn.

Table 4.2   Head to toe examination of newborn: normal and abnormal findings

Examination	Normal Findings	Abnormal Findings
Maturity	38–42 weeks	Prematurity, post maturity
Birth Weight	2500–4200 gms	Small for dates, large for dates
Birth length	45–55 cms	Too short, Abnormally short limbs
OFC	34–36 cm	Microcephaly, macrocephaly
Temp	37.0 C+/-0.5 C	Hypothermia, hyperthermia
Head	Shape may be influenced by moulding, caput succedaneum or in-utero position.	Vacuum extraction, haematoma, cephalhaematoma, subaponeurotic haemorrhage, depressed fracture
Fontanelle	Diamond shaped anterior, Triangular shaped posterior, rarely 2 lateral fontanelles	Fontanelles too big or too small
Sutures	1 sagittal, 2 coronal, 2 lambdoid sutures	Gross overriding or separation, premature closure
Face	Milia Normal appearance	Facial paralysis, coarse features
Eyes	Mild subconjunctival haemorrhage, blink reflex, pupils react to light	Discharge, excessive tearing, anaemia, jaundice before 24 hours, eyes too small or large, eyes widely spaced, epicanthic fold, cataract, abnormal blink or white light reflex

Ears	Normal position, responds to loud sound	Low set ears, congenital abnormalities like tag-or sinus, no response to loud sound
Nose	Nasal bridge flat, nostrils and nasal passages patent, nose breathing	Blockage, discharge, flaring alae nasi, and mouth breathing
Lips, jaw, oral cavity	Epstein pearls, sucking blisters, tongue tie	Cleft lip or palate, constant drooling, central cyanosis, small jaw
Neck	Short	Webbing, swellings, sinuses
Thorax	Cylindrical shape, physiological enlargement of breasts	Pectus excavatum, widely spaced nipples, hyperinflation, mastitis
Respiratory system	Respiratory rate 30– 50/m Quiet thoracic/abdominal breathing, expansion symmetrical, Air entry good, no adventitious sounds	Rate too slow or rapid, grunting, totally thoracic or abdominal breathing, expansion asymmetrical, overexpansion, intercostal, Subcostal, sternal retraction, apnoeic attacks, stridor, poor air entry, adventitious sounds
Cardiovascular system	Heart rate 100–160/m, Peripheral pulses palpable, Apex beat 4th left I.C. space, normal heart sounds	Bounding or weak pulses, absent femoral pulses, enlarged heart, thrills, murmurs

Skin	Vernix caseosa, Slight peripheral cyanosis, mongolian spots, milia, lanugo, erythema toxicum, capillary haemangioma	Gross desquamation, meconium staining, cyanosis, jaundice before 24 hours, deep jaundice any time, anaemia, plethora, petechiae, bruising, blisters, haemorrhage.
Central nervous system	Conscious but sleeps most of the time, cry normal, arms and legs semi-flexed, limb movements bilaterally present, tone symmetrical, Knees and biceps reflexes present and equal, planters extensor, cranial nerves all intact, follows bright light, responds to loud noise, primitive reflexes present e.g. sucking, rooting and moros	Irritability, high pitched cry, abnormal posture, persistent jitteriness, convulsions, lack or excessive movement, floppiness, hypertonic, Head retraction, reflexes unequal, absent or too brisk, eye rolling, eye deviation, setting sun sign, facial paralysis
The urine	More than 90% infants void within 24 hours	Dribbling, delayed urination, bladder distention.
The stools	Meconium passed within 36–48 hours	Delayed passage

CHAPTER 05

Respiratory System

- General Examination of Respiratory System
- Inspection
- Palpation
- Percussion
- Auscultation

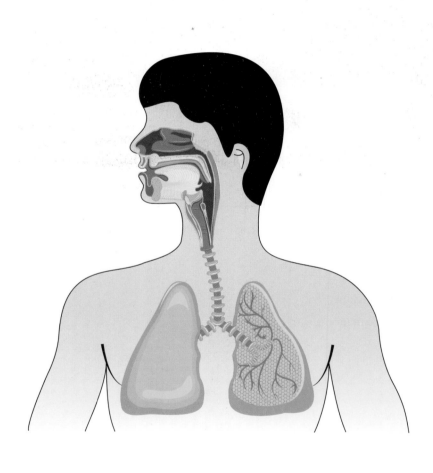

RESPIRATORY SYSTEM

Respiratory diseases are very common in paediatric age group especially below five. This is because of different reasons: small diameter of larynx, trachea and bronchi, immature respiratory immunological system, decrease surfactant formation, less compliant chest wall, and few fatigue resistant diaphragmatic muscles.

The sequence of respiratory examination depends upon the cooperation of the child. Ideally the child should be comfortably resting on a bed, sitting at the angle of 45 degree and supported by a pillow. Before examining the respiratory system, one should look for the sign of respiratory disease in general examination.

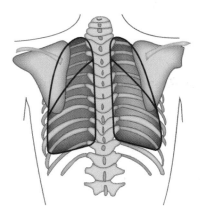

Fig. 5.1   Posterior chest

General Examination of Respiratory System

Look for signs of malnutrition and nature of the voice. The hands should be examined for clubbing, pallor or cyanosis. The lips and tongue should also be inspected for central cyanosis. Look for flaring alae nasi, use of accessory muscles of respiration, chest indrawing (Intercostal and subcostal) and palpate lymph nodes in the axilla, neck, and supraclavicular fossae.

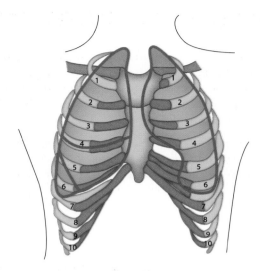

Fig. 5.2   Anterior chest

Examination of Respiratory System

Components of examination are:

- Inspection

- Palpation

- Percussion

- Auscultation

Most valuable part of examination especially during infancy is inspection. Palpation and percussion is not particularly a useful exercise in infants and toddlers.

INSPECTION

Apart from clubbing, cyanosis, flaring, chest indrawing and general nutritional status the two most important things during inspection of chest are shape of the chest and movements of the chest. The normal chest is bilaterally symmetrical and elliptical in cross section. Abnormalities in the shape of the chest is summarised in table 5.1.

Table 5.1   Abnormalities of shape of the chest.

Bulging
- Pleural effusion
- Pneumothorax
- Kyphosis
- Cardiomegaly
- Malunion of ribs

Retraction
- Collapse
- Fibrosis
- Pectus excavatum (sternal depression)
- Isolated congenital anomaly
- Chronic adenoidal hypertrophy

Bulging costochondral junction
- Rickets
- Scurvy

Barrel shaped chest
- Asthma
- Emphysema
- Other obstructive lung diseases

Miscellaneous
- Pre-sternal oedema (mumps)
- Hypoplastic nipples (Downs, Turner syndrome)

While observing the movement of the chest, one should note the rate, rhythm, type and symmetry of the chest movements. Asymmetrical expansion of the chest may occur when the underlying lung is abnormal e.g. pleural effusion, pneumothorax, consolidation, collapse or fibrosis.

The two most important abnormalities in the type of respiration are chyne stroke and kausmal breathing. The later is found in acidosis while the causes of former include severe pneumonia and narcotic drugs poisoning. Look also for movements of diaphragm. It is paralyzed in various disease especially poliomyelitis and Guillain barre syndrome. In case of diaphragmatic paralysis, bulging of abdomen occurs with respiration.

PALPATION

Note the following points:

Pain and Tenderness

It may be due to injury, inflammatory conditions, intercostal muscular pain, secondary malignant deposition, pleurisy, pericarditis etc.

Position of apex beat (See chapter on CVS examination).

Position of Trachea

Place index and ring finger to the right and left sterno-clavicular joint respectively, while the middle finger is free to feel the trachea. A slight deviation of the trachea to the right may be found in a healthy child. It is pulled when the lung is collapsed or fibrosed and pushed with pneumothorax or pleural effusion.

Chest Expansion

Place the finger tips of both hands on either side of the lower rib cage, so that tips of the thumbs meet in the midline. A deep breath will increase the distance between the thumbs and indicate the degree of expansion. It is decreased in lung and pleural pathology.

Tactile Vocal Fremitus

It can be easily assessed when the child is crying but this is not a commonly used routine technique of examination.

PERCUSSION

The sound and feel of resonance over a healthy lung has to be learnt by practise. One should systematically compare the percussion note on two equivalent sides of the chest. Compare three or four anterior and posterior areas of the chest and two or three areas in the lateral chest. The rules of percussion are summarised in table 5.2.

Percussion note is dull in collapse, consolidation, thickened pleura and fluid in the pleura cavity (stony dull). It is increased (Hyper-resonant) in pneumothorax, emphysema and above the level of pleural effusion.

Table 5.2   Rules of percussion

1.	Middle finger (pleximeter) of the left hand is placed on the part to be percussed.
2.	Back of the pleximeter (middle phalanx) is than struck with the tip of the middle finger of the right hand (Plexar).
3.	Movements should be at wrist.
4.	Terminal phalanx is at right angle to the metacarpal bone.
5.	Strike the pleximeter finger perpendicularly.
6.	Strike the plexar twice and then lift it off the pleximeter.
7.	Pleximeter should be perpendicular to the boarder of the organ to be percussed and it should be done from resonant to dull area.

Types of Percussion

1. Resonant e.g. lungs

2. Tympanitic e.g. stomach

3. Impaired e.g. junction of a solid organ

4. Dull e.g. solid organ

5. Stony dull e.g. fluid

AUSCULTATION

It is preferable to have paediatric stethoscope. It is smaller, warmer and applies better to the small chest. It allows less surface noise and is better attuned to receive low pitch chest sound. Care should also be taken that chest piece should not move on the skin. After having listened to the chest, the paediatrician should be able to comment on breath sounds, added sounds, and vocal resonance.

Breath Sound

Check the intensity and quality of the breath sound. The intensity (loudness) may be normal, decreased or increased. It is increased in very thin subjects and decreased if the lung is extensively damaged (emphysema), pleural thickening or pleural fluid. The quality of the breath sounds is described as either vesicular or bronchial. Vesicular breath sound is produced by passage of air though smaller airways.

This is soft, rustling in character and there is usually no pause between the end of inspiration and the beginning of expiration. In case of airway obstruction (e.g. asthma), the slowing of expiration prolongs the normal expiratory sound. Bronchial breath sound is produced by passage of air through larger airways. The sound resembles that obtained by listening over the trachea. Bronchial breathing is rather harsh and there is a gap before the expiratory sound is heard. This is present in case of consolidation, collapse or fibrosis.

Vocal Resonance

It can easily be tested in a crying child and compared on both the sides. In older children, ask him/her to say 'one, two, three' and then auscultate. Each point examined on one side of the chest should be compared at once with the corresponding point on the other side. Increased vocal resonance is called bronchophony as occur in consolidation, cavitation, collapse with patent bronchus and also above the level of pleural effusion. When words are heard clearly, as if the patient is speaking directly into the ear, is called whispering pectoriloquy.

Added Sounds

The following added sounds may arise in the lung or in the pleura.

Pleural Rub

Characteristic of pleural inflammation, usually associated with chest pain. It is rubbing in character, does not change in character after coughing and in some instance is palpable.

Wheeze

Musical sound associated with airway narrowing. Lower airway narrowing produces expiratory wheeze. The loudest most obvious wheeze is the stridor associated with laryngeal spasm or tracheal stenosis or upper airway obstruction. Wheeze may be localised (tumour, foreign body) called monophonic or generalised called polyphonic (asthma, bronchiolitis).

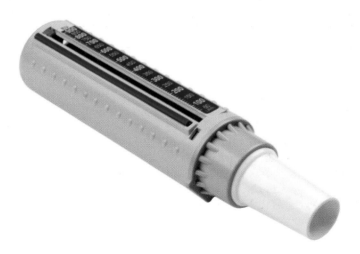

Fig. 5.3   Flow meter

Crackles: Short: explosive sound, described as bubbling or clicking noises. It may be expiratory in patients with airflow obstruction and may be inspiratory as in pulmonary oedema or with resolving pneumonia. The sounds are low pitched, scanty, loud and may clear with coughing.

Table 5.3 Physical features of common Lung pathology

	Movement	Percussion note	Breath sound	Vocal resonance
Consolidation	N	Dull	↓	↑
Collapse	↓	Dull	↓	↑
Pleural effusion	↓	Stony dull	↓	↓
Pneumothorax	↓	Hyper-resonant	↓	↓

'Until I was thirteen I thought my name was 'Shut up'.'

Joe Namath

'When I was a boy the Dead Sea was only sick.'

George Burns

CHAPTER 06

Cardiovascular System

- Examination of Precordium

  Inspection

  Palpation

  Auscultation

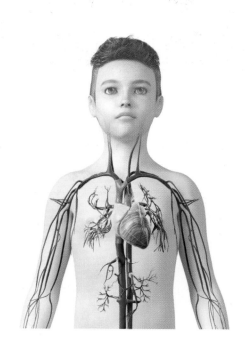

Cardiovascular System

Examine the cardiovascular system in the following order. Arterial pulse, blood pressure, venous pulse, precordium and auscultation. Before proceeding, the following general points should be noted:

- Dyspnoea with feeding
- Sweating
- Anaemia
- Oedema
- Central cyanosis
- Finger clubbing
- Splinter haemorrhage
- Breathlessness
- Hepatomegaly
- Splenomagaly

Arterial pulses, blood pressure and venous pulses: (described in chapter of general examination).

Examination of Precordium

INSPECTION

Look for the deformities of the chest wall. The presence of kyphosis, scoliosis or sternal depression should be noted. Sternal depression is sometimes associated with loud S-1, broad QRS complex, right bundle branch block and cardiac enlargement on X-ray chest.

Look for the pulsation in the precordium and outside the precordium especially in the neck, suprasternal notch, chest wall and epigastrium.

PALPATION

Palpate cardiac impulse i.e. apex beat, the lowest and outermost point of cardiac pulsation. Normally it is 9 cms from the midline or 1 cm medial to mid clavicular line in the fourth intercostal space. It should be noted in sitting or lying position. Causes of displacement of apex beat are pneumothorax, pleural effusion, collapse, fibrosis and ventricular hypertrophy. It is difficult to detect in Asthma, emphysema, pleural or pericardial effusion or obesity.

In pressure overload (aortic stenosis, systemic hypertension) there is forceful sustained heaving impulse while in volume overload (aortic or mitral regurgitation) there is equally forceful but less sustained impulse. During palpation of apex beat, also note thrill (palpable murmur), loud first sound (mitral stenosis) and loud second sound (systemic and pulmonary hypertension).

AUSCULTATION

It is important to identify correctly the systolic and diastolic periods. Palpation of the carotid artery provides a systolic time reference, so it is better to feel carotid artery while auscultation.

Following are the areas of auscultation

1. Mitral area at apex beat

2. Tricuspid area at left lower sternal border

3. Aortic area at upper right sternal border

4. Pulmonary area at upper left sternal border

Note the following points:

1. Normal heart sounds

2. Abnormal heart sounds

3. Extra-cardiac sounds

1. Normal Heart Sounds

First heart sound is produced due to the closure of tricuspid and mitral valve (M T). The closure of aortic and pulmonary valves produce second heart sound (AP).

2. Abnormal Heart Sounds

Following are considered as abnormal:

1. Different intensity of normal heart sounds (table 6.2)

2. Abnormal splitting (table 6.4)

3. Third or fourth heart sound (table 6.1)

4. Additional high pitch sound (table 6.3)

5. Murmur

First four are described in tables. Here murmur is described in detail:

Murmur

Turbulence in the blood flow at or near a valve or an abnormal communication within the heart may produce sound called murmur. Not all murmurs are produced by a structural disorder of the heart, such a murmur is called flow murmur. In examining a murmur the following points must be noted.

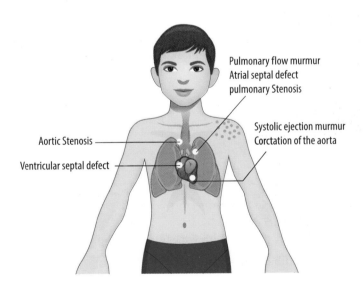

Fig. 6.1   Areas of murmur

Relation with cardiac cycle

Murmur may be systolic, diastolic, or continuous. It is better to feel the carotid artery during auscultation so that systole can be determined. Systolic murmur are either pansystolic (mitral or tricuspid regurgitation and ventricular septal defect), ejection systolic (pulmonary or systemic hypertension) or late systolic as is mitral valve prolapse. Diastolic murmurs are of two types, early diastolic (aortic or pulmonary regurgitation) and mid diastolic (mitral or tricuspid stenosis).

Location and radiation

Murmurs arising from tricuspid and pulmonary valves are well localised while aortic and mitral murmurs radiate extensively.

Relation with respiration

Generally a murmur originating from the right side of the heart will become louder during inspiration.

Character

Obstruction to flow through a narrow valve produces rough murmur while blowing murmur is more typical of an incompetent valve.

Intensity

Murmurs are graded as follow:

i.   Very soft

ii. Soft

iii. Loud without thrill

iv. Loud with thrill

v.   Loud with thrill, audible with edge of stethoscope

vi. Very loud, audible with naked ear

3. Extracardiac Sounds

Bruit and pericardial rub are the two most important extracardic sounds. Bruits are usually due to arterial stenosis, arising from a peripheral artery. A pericardial friction rub is a scratching noise produced by the movement of inflamed pericardium. It is high-pitched, best heard with diaphragm, obvious during systole and audible both in inspiration and expiration.

Table 6.1   Causes of third and fourth heart sounds

Third heart sound	Fourth heart sound
• Healthy young adult	• Pulmonary hypertension
• Left ventricular failure	• Systemic hypertension
• Mitral regurgitation	• Ischaemic heart disease
• Aortic regurgitation	

Table 6.2   Causes of change in intensity of heart sounds

Loud S 1	Decreased intensity of Sl
• Mitral stenosis	• Obesity
• Left ventricular failure	• Emphysema
• Atrial septal defect	• Pericardial effusion
• Left ventricular failure	• Pleural effusion
• Tachycardia	• Severe calcified mitral stenosis
• Left ventricular failure	• Mitral regurgitation
• Ebstein anomaly	• Heart failure

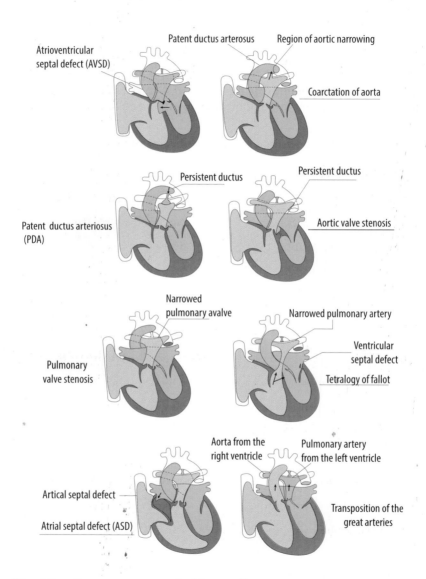

Fig. 6.2   Common congenital heart diseases

Cont.   Table 6.2

Loud S2	Decreased intensity of S2
• Left ventricular failure	• Calcified aortic stenosis
• Systemic hypertension	• Severe pulmonary hypertension
• Right ventricular failure	• Hypotension
• Pulmonary hypertension	

Table 6.3   Additional high pitched sounds

Ejection systolic click	Opening snap
• Congenital aortic stenosis	• Mitral stenosis
• Congenital pulmonary stenosis	• Tricuspid stenosis
• Pulmonary hypertension	
• Systemic hypertension	

Table 6.4   Causes of abnormal splitting

Wide splitting-mobile
• Pulmonary stenosis
• Right bundle branch block
• Pulmonary hypertension
• Ventricular septal defect
• Mitral regurgitation
• Pulmonary regurgitation
Wide splitting-fixed
• Atrial septal defect
Reversed splitting P2A2
• Left bundle branch block
• Hypertrophic cardiomyopathy
• Left ventricular failure
• Aortic stenosis

Table 6.5   Findings of common congenital heart diseases

	VSD	ASD	PDA	CA	TOF
Pulse	N	N	Bounding pulse	Radio femoral delay	N
Splitting	Wide mobile	Wide fixed	Narrow splitting	N	Single S-2
Murmur	PSM LLSB	ESM ULSB	Rough machinery ULSB	ESM	ESM ULSB
CXR	↑ PVM	↑ PVM	↑ PVM	Notching of ribs	↓ PVM
ECG	LVH (RVH When pul. Hypertension)	RAH RAD	LAH LVH	LVH	RVH

VSD-Ventricular Septal Defect, **ASD**-Atrial Septal Defect, **PDA**-Patent Ductus Arteriosus, **CA**-Coarctation of Aorta, **TOF**-Tetralogy of Fallots, **PSM**-Pansystolic Murmur, ESM-Ejection Systolic Murmur, **LLSB**-Lower Left Sternal Boarder, **ULSB**-Upper Left Sternal Boarder, **PVM**-Pulmonary Vascular Marking, **LVH**-Left Ventricular Hypertrophy, **RVH**-Right Ventricular Hypertrophy, **RAH**-Right Atrial Hypertrophy, **RAD**-Right Axis Deviation.

> 'An encyclopedia is a system for collecting dust in alphabetical order.'
>
> **Mike Barfield**

CHAPTER 07

Abdominal Examination

- General signs of Abdominal Disease
- Inspection
- Palpation
- Percussion
- Auscultation

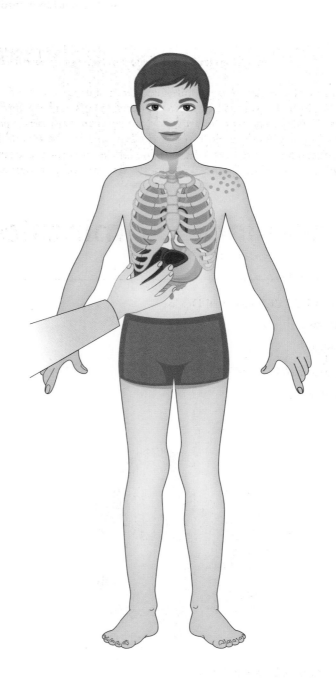

Abdominal Examination

Examination of the abdomen requires cooperation from the child. The patient should lie flat on his back, arms by his side and head is supported by pillows. The abdomen is divided into nine parts by two lateral vertical lines crossing the tip of the ninth costal cartilage and two horizontal lines namely subcostal and intercristal lines (figure 7.2) before proper abdominal examination, one should note the general features of gastrointestinal disease.

General Signs of Abdominal Disease

Note the following important points:

1. Signs of malnutrition
2. State of hydration
3. Clubbing
4. Jaundice
5. Anthropometric measurement

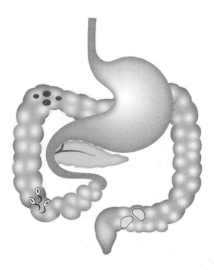

Fig. 7.1   Gastrointestinal tract

Inflammatory bowel disease often presents with extra-intestinal manifestations e.g. arthritis, uveitis and skin rashes including erythema nodosum and pyoderma gangrenosum.

INSPECTION

Should be done in good light, on the right side and ensure your hands are warm. Expose abdomen from xiphisternum to upper thigh and note the following:

Shape

Is it normal, distended or sunken. Sunken abdomen is seen in malnutrition, dehydration or severe illness. Distention may be due to the fat, flatus, faeces, fluid, viceromegaly or muscle hypotonia.

Umbilicus

Note its position, shape, hernia, drainage or mass.

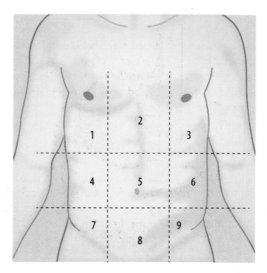

Fig. 7.2   Parts of Abdomen.

Visible Peristalsis

It may be seen in pyloric stenosis, duodenal atresia, paralytic ileus, volvulus, malrotation etc.

Skin

Look for any scar, pigmentations, superficial vein or striae. Check the direction of blood flow when veins are prominent. This will be demonstrated by pressing the vein with two fingers held close together, now empty the vein by separating the fingers. Release one finger and see if the vein fills, if it does not, release other finger to see if the emptied vein fills. In case of inferior caval obstruction, the direction of blood flow is from below upward.

Movements

It is restricted in peritonitis or in appendicitis. Paradoxical movement i.e. bulging with respiration, is seen in the case of paralysis of diaphragm e.g. poliomyelitis and Guillain-Barre syndrome.

PALPATION

The technique of abdominal palpation is an art. This will require patience, skill and distraction techniques. You may occasionally have to palpate the abdomen with the infant crawling. Some toddlers allow palpating while standing. Crying children relax the abdominal muscle during inspiration, permitting a brief period when palpation is possible.

Superficial Palpation

It is done to check tenderness, guarding, and mass. It is done by placing right hand flat on the abdomen in the left iliac fossa with the wrist and forearm in the same horizontal plane. Feel with slight flexion at the metacarpophalangeal joints, work anti-clockwise to end in the suprapubic region.

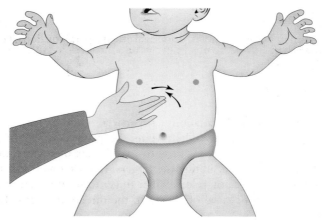

Fig. 7.3   Method of palpating liver

Liver (Fig. 7.3)

Place both hands side by side flat on the abdomen in right sub-costal region with fingers pointing towards the ribs. At the height of inspiration press the fingers firmly inward and upward to feel the liver. A liver 1–2 cms below the right costal margin is considered normal up to the age of 2–3 years. The causes and mechanism of liver enlargement is described in table 7.1. Alternate method of palpating liver is from radial border of the right index finger as described in figure 7.2.

Table 7.1   Common causes of hepatomegaly

- **Storage disorder:**

  Malnutrition, obesity, (total parenteral nutrition), cystic fibrosis, diabetes mellitus

  Gaucher, Niemann-pick, Wolman syndromes Alpha 1 antitrypsin deficiency, Wilson disease

- **Infections:**

  Viral-acute and chronic hepatitis

  Bacterial (sepsis, abscess, cholangitis, enteric fever)

  Protozoal (Malaria, leishmaniasis)

- **Autoimmune**

Chronic hepatitis, sarcoidosis, systemic lupus erythematosus, sclerosing cholangitis

- **Primary infiltration**

  Primary tumours

  Hepatoblastoma

  Hepatocellular carcinoma

  Hemangioma

  Focal nodular hyperplasia

- **Secondary or metastatic tumours**

  Lymphoma

  Leukaemia

  Histocytosis

  Neuroblastoma

  Wilms tumour

- **Increased size of Vascular Space**

  Veno-occlusive disease

  Hepatic vein thrombosis (Budd-Chiari syndrome)

  Congestive heart failure

  Pericardial disease

  Constrictive pericarditis

- **Increased size of Biliary Space**

  Congenital hepatic fibrosis

  Caroli disease

  Extrahepatic obstruction

- **Idiopathic ('Benign')**

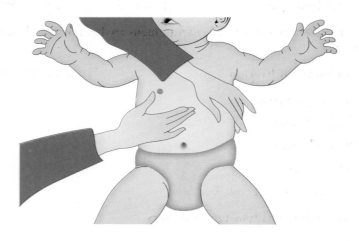

Fig. 7.4   Method of palpating spleen.

Table 7.2   Common causes of splenomegaly

Infection	
Bacterial:	Typhoid fever, endocarditis, septicaemia, abscess
Viral:	Epstein-Barr, cytomegalovirus, and others
Protozoal:	Malaria, toxoplasmosis
Hematologic Processes	
Haemolytic anaemia:	Congenital and acquired
Extramedullary hematopoiestis:	Thalassaemia, osteopetrosis, myelofibrosis
Neoplasms	
Malignant:	Leukaemia, lymphoma, metastatic disease

Benign:	Haemangioma, hamartoma
Infiltration and storage diseases	
Lipidoses:	Niemann-Pick, gaucher diseases
Mucopolysaccharidosis histiocytosis	
Congestion	
Cirrhosis or hepatic fibrosis hepatic, portal or splenic vein obstruction Congestive heart failure	
Cysts	
Congenital (true cysts) Acquired (pseudocysts)	
Miscellaneous	
Lupus erythematosus, sarcoidosis, rheumatoid arthritis	

Spleen (Figure 7.4)

Place the flat of the left hand over the lowermost rib cage postereolaterally and the right hand beneath the costal margin. Press deeply the fingers of the right hand beneath the costal margin, at the same time exerting pressure medially and downward with the left hand. When spleen is palpable, distinguish it from enlarged kidney. Distinguishing points of enlarged spleen from enlarged kidney are:

1. Dull to percuss

2. Not bimanually palpable

3. Upper border cannot be felt

4. Anterior border notched

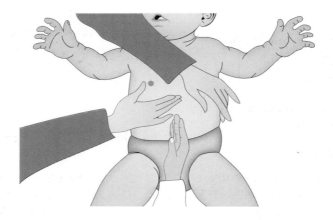

Fig. 7.5   Fluid thrill.

Kidneys

Place right hand anteriorly in the lumber region and left hand posteriorly in the loin. Feel while pressing the left hand forward and right hand backward, upwards and inwards. The lower pole of the right kidney is commonly palpable as smooth rounded swelling which descends with respiration and is bimanually palpable. Causes of enlargement of kidney are wilms tumour, renal vein thrombosis, polycystic disease, hydronephrosis, congenital nephrosis, multicystic dysplasia etc.

Urinary Bladder

It is an abdominal organ in neonates and early infancy. It becomes abdominal in older children when distended. It is felt in the suprapubic area as a symmetrical oval shaped swelling, firm in consistency, smooth surface with a regular margin. Causes of distended bladder are poliomyelitis, GB syndrome, acute transverse myelitis, obstructive uropathy etc.

Miscellaneous

Palpate aorta, femoral artery, para aortic lymph nodes and inguinal lymph nodes

Genitalia

Look for labial adhesions, clitoromegaly, perineal excoriation, vaginal discharge (female). Size and shape of penis, position of testis, hydrocele, hypospadiasis, balanitis (male) etc.

PERCUSSION

Method and rules of percussion are described in chapter of respiratory examination.

Only light percussion is necessary in abdomen. A tympanitic note is heard throughout the abdomen except over liver. Percussion is done to map out the organs accurately and to detect the ascites. Two signs, shifting dullness and fluid thrill, which present either singly or together, make the diagnosis of ascites certain.

Shifting Dullness

Percuss laterally from the midline, in a supine patient, keeping your fingers in the longitudinal axis, until dullness is detected. In normal individuals, it is detected at the lateral abdominal wall. Keep the hand over this area and roll the patient away to the opposite side. Purcuss again, if dull note becomes resonant then ascetic fluid is probably present.

Fluid Thrill (Figure 7.5)

Tap the lumbar region while placing one hand flat over the lumbar region of the opposite side. Get an assistant to put the side of the hand firmly in the midline. A fluid thrill or wave is felt by the detecting hand held flat in the lumbar region. A purpose of assistant is to prevent transmission of impulse through fat. Causes of ascites are described in table 7.3

AUSCULTATION

Bowel sounds are normally audible, just below and right to the umbilicus. It is accentuated if there is an increase in peristalsis e.g. diarrhoea and mechanical obstruction. It can be sluggish or absent in case of ileus.

Table 7.3   Common causes of ascites

Cardiac causes
- Constrictive pericarditis
- Congestive cardiac failure

Renal causes
- Nephrotic syndrome
- Acute renal failure

Hepatic causes
- Chronic hepatitis
- Acute fulminant hepatic failure

Venous causes
- Budd–Chiari syndrome
- Portal vein obstruction
- Inferior venacaval obstruction

Miscellaneous
- Lymphatic obstruction
- Beri Beri
- Meigs syndrome
- Tuberculous peritonitis
- Protein losing enteropathy
- Kwashiorkor

'Civilization is a limitless multiplication of unnecessary necessities.'

Mark Twain

'Good teachers are costly, but bad teachers cost more.'

Robert Talbert

'If you cannot convince them, confuse them.'

Harry S. Truman

CHAPTER 08

Central Nervous System

- State of Consciousness
- Position
- Memory
- Speech
- Fontanelle
- Cranial Nerves
- Motor System
- Sensory System
- Reflexes
- Sign of Meningeal Irritation

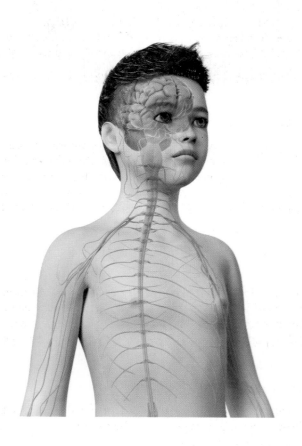

Central Nervous System

Detailed neurological examination is not described here. In older children it is conducted in the same way as in adults. Brief outlines are given with emphasis on CNS evaluation in infants, toddlers, and preschool children.

Following sequence is followed while examining central nervous system:

1. State of Consciousness

Normal components of appearance include awareness, responsiveness, activity and orientation. A comatose child is unresponsive and unaware but a paralyzed child is unresponsive but aware. A newly proposed classification of coma eliminates old words such as coma, semi coma, coma vigil, stupor etc. This is called Glasgow coma scale or EMV-Scale, described in table 8.1.

2. Position

Note the position deviated from normal e.g. opisthotonic (incurving back), decerebrate (extension of all four limbs), decorticate (extension of lower limbs and flexion of upper limbs). Look also for facial palsy, wrist drop, or erb's palsy. The child with severe hypotonia is in a pithed frog position.

3. Memory

Say 1, 2, 3 and ask the child to repeat 1, 2, 3 and then 3, 2, 1 (short term memory). To test long-term memory, ask the child about his home address, birth date and names and ages of siblings.

4. Speech

Check for the presence or absence of speech, quality of speech, and quantity of speech (age-appropriate). Failure to speak any word by 18 months and failure to make meaningful sentences by 3 years are abnormal. Complete absence of speech is mutism and may be an evidence of deafness, mental retardation, or autism.

Table 8.1   Glasgow coma scale

Eye Opening

NO.	> 1 YEAR	< 1 YEAR
4	Spontaneously	Spontaneously
3	To verbal command	To shout
2	To pain	To pain
1	No response	No response

Best Motor Response

NO.	> 1 YEAR	< 1 YEAR
6	Obeys	Spontaneously
5	Localises pain	Localises pain
4	Flexion: Withdrawal	Flexion: Withdrawal
3	Flexion: Abnormal decorticate rigidity	Flexion: Abnormal decerebrate rigidity
2	Extension: Decerebrate rigidity	Extension: Decerebrate rigidity
1	No response	No response

Best Verbal Response

NO.	> 5 YEAR	2–5 YEAR	< 1 YEAR
5	Oriented and converses	Appropriate words	Smiles, coos
4	Disoriented and converses	Inappropriate words	Cries: consolable

3	Inappropriate words	Presistent Cry or Screams	Persistent Inappropriate Cry or Screams
2	Incomprehensible sounds	Grunts	Grunts: Agitated or restless
1	No response	No response	No response

5. Fontanelle

Anterior fontanelle is 2.5 x 2.5 cms in size. It is usually closed at 9–18 months of age. Posterior fontanelle is very small at birth and closes rapidly by two months of age. Examination of anterior fontanelle is summarised in table 8.2.

Table 8.2   Interpretation of anterior fontanelle

Closes too early	Microcephaly, craniosynostosis
Wide/Delayed closure	Hypothyroidism, hydrocephalus, rickets, malnutrition, dawn syndrome etc.
Tense or Elevated	Increased intracranial pressure
Depressed	Sign of dehydration

6. Cranial Nerves

It is difficult to examine cranial nerves in infants and young children, although with practise observation of child on movements may enable a partial examination to be made. For example eye movements (3, 4, 6) chewing (5), crying, smiling (7), sucking (5, 7, 9), swallowing (9, 10, 11), phonation (9, 10), head turning (11), tongue protrusion (12). Non functioning cranial nerves are also assessed by observations e.g. loss of vision (2), squint, diplopia, deconjugate movements of eye (3,4,6) loss of facial sensation and corneal reflex (5), sign of facial palsy (7), failure to respond normal sounds or delayed speech (8), stridor, hoarse voice, nasal regurgitation, loss of palatal reflex and gag reflex (9,10), unable to shrug shoulder (11) and unable to protrude tongue (12).

7. Motor System

Following points should be noted during examination of motor system. Bulk, tone, strength, coordination, involuntary movements, reflexes and gait. Differential diagnosis of upper motor neuron paralysis and lower motor neuron paralysis are described in table 8.5.

a. Bulk

Look for muscle wasting and atrophy, observe symmetry and asymmetry of wasting. Proximal wasting seen in myopathies and malabsorbtion and distal wasting seen in peripheral neuritis.

Also check muscle hypertrophy. It may be hemihypertrophy (congenital), psuedohypertrophy (Duchenne muscular dystrophy) or true hypertrophy (exercise). Always compare the two sides of the body.

b. Tone

State of tension or resistance to passive movement is called tone. It is decreased (hypotonia) in lower motor neuron lesion, hypothyroidism, down syndrome, cerebellar lesion etc. and increased (hypertonia) in upper motor neuron lesion, anxiety,spastic type of cereberal palsy and lesion of basal ganglion. Tone is assessed by passive movement of flexion and extension in all four limbs.

c. Strength

Ideally it is tested by asking the child to bring muscle into action against the resistance offered by the doctor. In children it is not always possible, therefore some simple tests for important muscles should be done as rapid screening. For example, ask the patient to get up from supine position (neck flexors), to elevate arm above the head (deltoid), to flex the elbow (biceps), to extend arm against resistance (triceps), to flex and abduct the hip (gluteus medius), to lift hip off the table (back muscle), to push examiner's palm with sole of the foot (gastrocnemius and soleus) etc. Grading of weakness is described in Table 8.3.

Table 8.3   Grading of weakness

0.	Complete paralysis
1.	Flicker of contraction
2.	Power observed when gravity excluded
3.	Against force of gravity not against examiner's resistance
4.	Some degree of weakness (moderate strength)
5.	Normal power

d. Coordination

For proper coordination of muscle movement the muscle must be strong, agonist and antagonist should act together and normal functioning of cerebellum. Coordination of upper limbs is assessed by finger-finger test (ask the child to touch the index fingers of both hand with closed eye in front of chest), finger-nose test (ask to touch nose with index finger) and making a circle in the air. Coordination of lower limbs is checked by heel knee test (ask to touch shin with the heel of opposite leg, down to its whole length) and to walk along a straight line. Other method for checking coordination of movements includes riding a cycle, making a circle, tying button or shoes laces, writing or drawing a person etc.

e. Involuntary Movements

There are many types of abnormal movements that are involuntary. The most important being described here:

i. Tics

Purposeless, repetitive movement usually involves face, eye and upper limbs.

ii. Chorea

Purposeless, non-repetitive, usually associated with hypotonia and poor coordination.

iii. Myoclonus

Intermittent contractions of a single muscle or groups of muscles.

iv. Athetosis

Slow rhythmic movements commonly involve distal muscles.

v. Dystonia

Fluctuation in tone usually involves the proximal muscles and disappears during sleep.

f. Reflexes

(Detailed descriptions in next section)

g. Gait

This is a part of neurological examination in older children. Following abnormal types of gait may be seen:

i. Spastic gait

Difficulty in bending knee as child steps forward, raises his hip up and swings in a semicircular fashion. It is seen in spastic type of cerebral palsy and lesion of pyramidal tract.

ii. Scissor gait

Legs will cross each other while walking. It is seen in cerebral palsy and slipped femoral epiphyses.

iii. Waddling gait

Body sways more or less from side to side. It indicates congenital dislocation of hip joint or myopathy

iv. Ataxic gait

A broad base or drunken gait seen in cerebellar lesion, drugs or tick-bite paralysis.

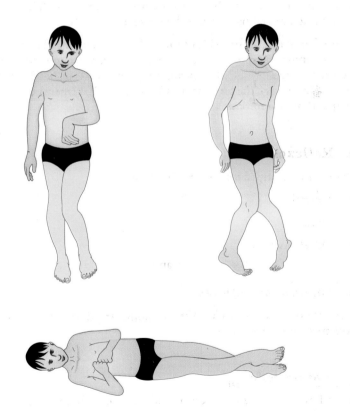

Fig. 8.1   Abnormal gaits and posture.

5. Sensory System

The sensations are classified under four headings;

- Superficial: Pain, touch, and temperature.
- Deep: Pressure, vibration and joint sensation.
- Cortical: Stereognosis, and discrimination .
- Special sensation: Smell, taste, hearing and vision.

The sensory system is very difficult to examine in children and can be tested only in older children. In infants the crying or withdrawal response to pin prick can be used to test the sensation crudely.

Loss of sensation on one side of the body is rare and may be seen following a head injury. Hyperasthesia is seen in transverse myelitis, peripheral neuritis, herpes zoster and during recovery phase of head injury etc. In spinal cord injury, the level of anesthesia has to be remembered in relation to the injured vertebrae.

6. Reflexes

Reflexes are grouped under three headings:

1. Superficial
2. Deep
3. Developmental

a. Superficial Reflexes

The main reflexes under this heading includes planter, cremestric abdominal and anal reflex.

i. Planter reflex

Scratching along the outer border of the foot with blunt object, produce planter flexion of great toe and flexion and adduction of other toes. Abnormal planter reflex (dorsiflexion) indicate pyramidal lesion.

ii. Cremesteric reflex

Stroking of upper medical thigh produces contraction of cremesteric muscle with elevation of the scrotum. It is lost in lesion above L2.

iii. Abdominal reflex

Contraction of the abdominal wall at the stimulated quadrant, as shown by the movement of the umbilicus towards stimulant. Its absence indicate upper motor neuron lesion.

iv. Anal reflex

Pricking of perianal skin, causes contraction of the external anal sphincter. Abnormality indicates lesion involving S2–4.

b. Deep Reflexes

i. Biceps reflex

Flex the elbow and thumb of the supported hand is held over biceps. Thumb is then tapped with hammer and note the contraction of the biceps (C5–6).

ii. Triceps reflex

A sharp tap over triceps tendon when elbow is flexed and forearm is supported by examiner, will produce contraction of triceps muscle (C6–8).

iii. Brahioradialis

Tap the styloid process of radius, when forearm is slightly flexed and between pronation and supination. Normal response is flexion and supination of forearm (C6–7).

iv. Knee jerk

When child lying supine, the knees are supported by examiners hand and flexed. Tap the patellar tendon and note the contraction of quadriceps muscle (L2–L4); It can also be elicited when patient is sitting at the edge of the bed with the knee hanging free.

v. Ankle jerk

It is tested in various positions but the best position is prone with flexed knee and hold the toes down firmly and tap the achilles tendon. Normal response is planter flexion (Sl-2).

c. Developmental Reflexes

In the natural course of development, spinal cord reflexes are present at birth and persist up to 2 weeks. Brain stem reflexes appear at this time and should disappear by the six months. Midbrain reflexes start appearing at 4–6 months and persist up to two years when cortical reflexes appear. Persistence of these reflexes or reappearance after normal progression may suggest some brain insult. Table 8.4 highlights the brief descriptions about these reflexes. Details are given in chapter of neonatal examination.

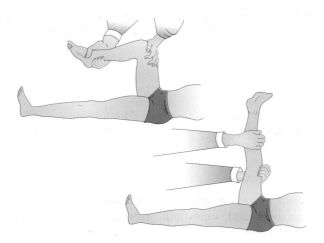

Fig. 8.2   Kerning's sign.

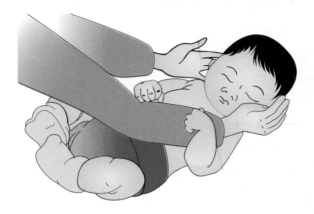

Fig. 8.3   Method of eliciting neck rigidity.

6.   Signs of Meningeal Irritation

a.   Neck Rigidity (Figure 8.3)

Ask to flex the chin, to kiss the knee or to look at the roof. If the child cannot do all the above readily, neck rigidity is likely to be present. It can also be checked by active method and observe the infants position of comfort.

b.   Kernings Sign (Figure 8.2)

Flex the hip and knee to right angle and slowly extend the leg. In case of positive sign there is pain and limitation of movement.

c.   Brudzinkis Sign

Flexion of head produces flexion of both knee and thigh (head method), and flexion of one leg causes flexion of other leg (leg method).

Table 8.4   Development reflexes

Spinal cord reflexes
• Flexor withdrawal
• Extensor thrust
• Cross extensor reflex
Brain stem reflexes
• Asymmetric tonic neck reflex
• Symmetrical tonic neck reflex
• Positive supporting reaction
• Negative supporting reaction
• Tonic labyrinthine reflex
Mid-brain reflexes
• Neck on body righting
• Labyrinthine righting
• Optical righting
Cortical reflexes
• Hoping reflex
• Placing (adult type) reflex

Table 8.5   Differential diagnosis of upper and lower motor neuron paralysis

Feature	UMN paralysis	LMN paralysis
Bulk and nutrition	No wasting	Marked wasting
Power	Groups of muscles are involved	Individual muscles are involved
Tone	Increased	Decreased
Tendon jerks	Brisk	Diminished or absent
Plantar	Up going (Babinski's sign is positive)	Down going (Babinski's sign is negative)
Abdominal and cremasteric reflexes	Absent	Present (these are absent if concerned spinal roots or nerves are affected)
Fasciculations	Absent	May be present

'It is now proved beyond doubt that smoking is one of the leading causes of statistics.'

Fletcher Knebel

CHAPTER 09

Examination of the Head

- Inspection
- Palpation
- Percussion
- Auscultation
- Transillumination

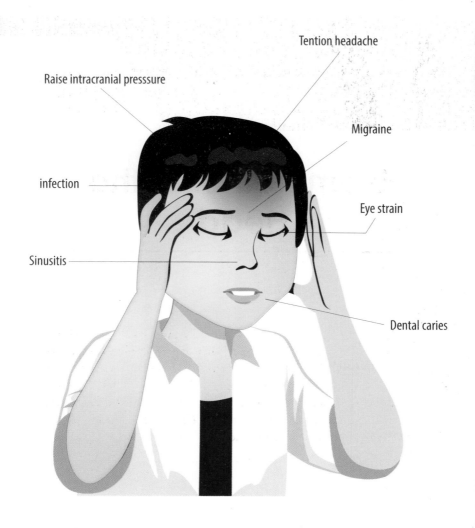

Tention headache

Raise intracranial presssure

Migraine

infection

Eye strain

Sinusitis

Dental caries

Common causes of Headache

Examination of the Head

Examination of head should be done under following methods:

1. Inspection

2. Palpation

3. Percussion

4. Auscultation

5. Transillumination

INSPECTION

Following points should be noted while inspecting the head:

Size

The measurement techniques and the normal growth pattern is given in the chapter of general examination under the heading of physical parameters. Head circumference (OFC) greater than two standard deviations over the mean for age, sex, race and gestation is called macrocephaly. Similarly when the OFC is two standard deviation below the mean for age, sex, race and gestation, than it is called microcephaly. The causes of macrocephaly and microcephaly are described in table 9.1.

Shape

Note any asymmetry in the skull shape. Asymmetrical skulls are caused by inequality of growth rates at the coronal, sagittal and lambdoid sutures. The inequality may be due to the following reasons:

• Postural effect: Infant who lies in one position only.

• Premature fusion of the sutures known as craniosynostosis. Causes of cranoisynostosis includes certain inherited syndromes, metabolic disorders such as hypophosphatasia and idiopathic.

It is also reported after excessive thyroxine therapy (see table 9.2).

Table 9.1   Causes of macrocephaly and microcephaly

Macrocephaly	Microcephaly
Hydrocephalus	**Genetic causes**
Achondroplasia	Inherited as autosomal
Osteopetrosis	Recessive trait.
Rickets	**Trisomy syndrome.**
Neurocutaneous syndrome	**Pelvic irradiation**
Tuberousclerosis	**Intrauterine infection**
Neurofibromatosis	Rubella
Metabolic diseases	Syphilis
Leucodystrophies	Toxoplasmosis
Mucopolysaccharidosis	Cytomegalovirus
Subdural haematoma	**Postnatal asphyxia**
Sotos syndrome	**Malnutrition in early infancy**
(cerebral gigantism).	

Table 9.2   Types of craniosynostosis

Scaphocephaly or Dolicocephaly	Premature closure of sagittal suture The head expand in anteroposterior direction
Brachycephaly	Premature closure of coronal suture causing broadening of skull with short anteroposterior diameter
Trigonocephaly	Forehead appears pointed and ridged due to premature closure of metopic suture.
Oxycephaly or Turricephaly	Involvement of all sutures.

Frontal Bossing

Rounded prominences in the frontal region found in infants with rickets. Sometimes it is familial.

Hair

The quality of the hair, its shine, thickness, fineness, coarseness, pluckability and discolouration should be noted.

Areas of alopecia should be mentioned.

PALPATION

Three important areas should be palpated.

Fontanelles

It is described in the chapter of Central Nervous System.

Sutures

The suture lines are not normally palpable after six months. Final closure does not occur until after adult life with the exception of metopic suture that closes in neonatal life. Premature closure of sutures results in various cranial deformities as described in the shape of the head.

Craniotabes

It is felt by pressing the skull firmly with the fingers (slightly separated) just above and behind the ears eliciting a ping-pong ball sensation. It indicates softening of the outer table of skull. Normal below six months. It is also seen in rickets, syphilis and hydrocephalus.

PERCUSSION

A cracked pot percussion note (Macewen's sign) is elicited by tapping the skull particularly with one finger, not far away from the suture line.

A hollow note is heard if the sutures are separated by space occupying lesions but such sound is normally heard if fontanelle is open. It is of some significance after the closure of fontanelles and indicates increased intracranial pressure or dilated ventricle.

AUSCULTATION

Findings of intracranial bruits on auscultation of skull and orbits should be sought. It occurs in region of vascular malformation, tumours and space occupying lesion that may compress large vessel.

Cranial bruits are commonly heard in normal infants and young children. 60% of 4–5 years of age. 10% of 10 years old children. So one should be cautious in their interpretation.

TRANSILLUMINATION

Transillumination is a valuable examination technique. It is done by chungun transilluminater or flashlight. The procedures should be carried out in a dark room after the examiner has adapted to darkness. It is sometimes helpful in diagnosis of hydrocephalus.

'Logic is a systematic method of coming to the wrong conclusion with confidence.'

Manly's Maxim

'A study of economics usually reveals that the best time to buy anything is last year.'

Marty Allen

Examination of the Neck

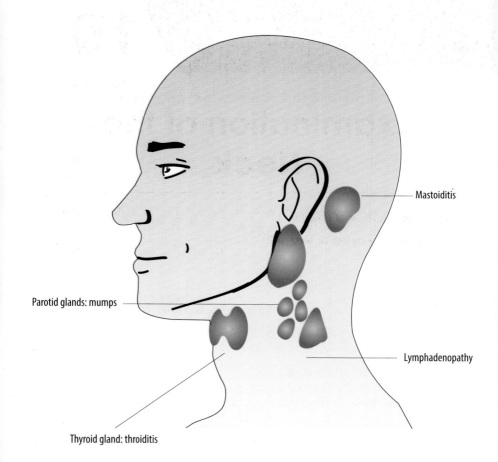

Mastoiditis

Parotid glands: mumps

Lymphadenopathy

Thyroid gland: throiditis

Common causes of neck swelling

Examination of the Neck

Look for presence of any swelling, sinuses, thyroid enlargement, lymph node enlargement, JVP, salivary glands and tenderness (see chapter of general examination.) Examination of neck may give clues to some diseases. Few examples are given below:

- The neck is short in infancy. Short neck in children is seen in Hurler syndrome, Hypothyroidism, Sprangel deformity, Down syndrome etc.

- Neck is long and thin in Marfan syndrome and some types of myopathy (Swan neck).

- Thyrogolossal duct, cysts or fistulas may be located in the midline of the neck, anywhere from the root of the neck to the suprasternal notch.

- Branchial fistulas usually open along the anterior border of the mastoid muscle.

- Swelling of the neck occurs in lymphadenopathy (most common), cystic hygroma, lipomas.

- Torticollis (wry neck). see table 10.2

- Webbing of the neck is seen in Turner's syndrome

- Laxity of the skin about the neck may be present in children with Cutis laxa, Pseudo Xanthoma elastica, Down syndrome, Turner syndrome etc.

- Observation of vessels in the neck (both arterial and venous) provides useful information. See chapter of C.V.S. examination.

- Thyroid enlargement (goiter) may be obvious on inspection. It moves with deglutition. In patients with hyperthyroidism, bruits and palpable thrill can be elicited. Classification of goiter is described in table 10.1.

Table 10.1   Classification of Goiter

Grading	Explanation
I-A	Palpable
I-B	Visible with tilted neck
II	Visible with normal neck position
III	Visible from 10 meters

Table 10.2   Common causes of Torticollis

• Congenital muscular torticollis	• Upper lobe pneumonia
• Acquired muscular injury	• Cervical lymphadenitis
• Dystonic drug reaction	• Cervical vertebral osteomyelitis
• Posterior fossa tumour	• Retropharyngeal abscess
• Benign paroxysmal torticollis	• Rheumatoid arthritis

'We spend the first twelve months of our children's lives teaching them to walk and talk and the next twelve telling them to sit down and shut up.'

Phyllis Diller

CHAPTER 11

Examination of the Eyes

- General Examination
  - Orbit
  - Cornea and Conjunctiva
  - Sclera
  - Red-eye reflex
- Neurological Examination
  - Cortical Vision
  - Pupil
  - Visual acuity
  - Visual field
  - Ocular movements
  - Opthalmoscopy

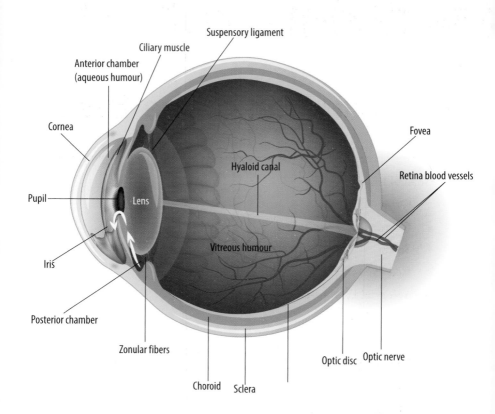

Suspensory ligament

Ciliary muscle

Anterior chamber
(aqueous humour)

Cornea

Fovea

Retina blood vessels

Pupil

Lens

Hyaloid canal

Iris

Vitreous humour

Posterior chamber

Zonular fibers

Choroid

Sclera

Optic disc

Optic nerve

Examination of the Eyes

Examination of eyes comprises two components.

1. General examination
2. Neurological examination

General Examination

(summarised in Table 11.1)

Table 11.1 General examination of eyes (check list):

Orbit
• Size of eyes
• Ptosis (Table11.2)
• Puffiness of eyelids
• Proptosis
• Epicanthic folds
• Sunken eye
• Hypertelorism
Cornea and Conjunctiva
• Corneal haziness(Table 11.3)
• Keratitis
• Keratomalacia
• Conjunctivitis
• Haemorrhage
• Corneal ulceration
• Xerosis.

Sclera

- Colour of Sclera
- Jaundice
- Bitot spots
- Xerosis(dryness)
- Kayser fleischer ring

Check red-eye reflex (Table 11.4)

Table 11.2   Causes of Ptosis

- Lesion of third nerve
- Horner syndrome
- Congenital (aut.dominant)
- Mysthenia gravis
- Botulism

Table 11.3   Causes of Corneal opacity

- Keratitis
- Vitamin A deficiency
- Hurler syndrome

Table 11.4   Causes of white eye reflex-leukocoria

- Retinoblastoma
- Retrolental fibroplasia
- Toxocariasis
- Cataract

- Corneal opacity
- Retinal detachment

Table 11.5   Common causes of Cataract

• Hereditary	• Steroid toxicity
• Developmental	• Hypocalcemia
• Prematurity	• Neonatal hypoglycemia
• TORCH infections	• Diabetes mellitus
• Galactosemia	• Mucopolysaccharidosis
• Trisomies	• Wilson disease

Table 11.6   Causes of Mydriasis

- Fear or anxiety
- 3rd nerve palsy
- Hippocampus herniation
- Atropine toxicity
- Pinealoma

Table 11.7   Causes of Miosis

- Pontine haemorrhage
- Deep coma
- Horner syndrome
- Pilocarpine toxicity
- Organophosphorus poisoning

Neurological Examination of the Eyes

Cortical Vision

Following things can be noted to assess the intact vision:

- Consistent blinking
- Follows moving object or light
- Response to bright light

Pupil

- Check shape, size and equality of both pupils.
- Pupillary response to light, pain and accommodation.
- Causes of constricted and dilated pupil are described in Table 11.6 and 11.7.

Visual Acuity

In infants and children always ask the mother. Can your child see well? She replies yes, ask her 'Tell me why do you think so?' If she is worried about the baby's vision, take her word for it. She is usually right. Some warning signs of poor visual acuity in early infancy are:

1. Roving or wandering eye movements.
2. Persistence of hand regard
3. Lack of blinking movements
4. Nystygmus

Visual acuity is best tested by grading the patient's ability to identify symbols decreasing in size (snellen's chart) usually by the age of 4 years. E symbols and pictures are commonly used for non-cooperative child. The child is taught to point his finger in the direction as the fingers of the E.

Below the age of six months, vision may be assessed by noting the childs interest in a bright object, whether child fixes a gaze on familiar object like toys.

Visual Field

Peripheral vision can be tested for gross defects by using confrontation method. The patient and the examiner face each other about one meter apart. Then for example the right eye of the patient and the left eye of the examiner are closed and they fixate each other open eyes. Then examiner using his own visual field, he moves first object (small white head pins or his finger) inward from the periphery and note when they are first seen by the patients. Each quadrant of each eye is checked separately. This confrontation test can only be done in cooperative children.

Ocular Movements

Check the eye movements in all four directions (inward, outward, upward and downward). External squint is seen in third nerve palsy while abducent nerve palsy may have internal squint.

Ophthalmoscopy

Good ophthalmoscopy is an integral part of the examination of any child irrespective of age.

In the newborn period it is easily performed, only an assistance is required to hold the head correctly in the mid line. The eyelids can be generally pressed apart.

Checklist of Ophthalmoscope

• Elicit the red reflex in both the eyes at a distance of 20 cms. The common causes of white eye reflex are described in Table 11.4

• Inspect cornea for clarity.

• Look at the lens for opacity (Table 11.5).

• Examine the fundus to detect haemorrhages, exudates, vessels, pigmentary changes and appearance of disc.

• Check the size of the eyes if they are too big (glaucoma) or too small (micropthalmus).

It is difficult to perform ophthalmoscopy in toddlers and pre-school children. Do not try to forcibly open the eye by pressing the lids apart.

This is invariably unsuccessful. Make the child and infant in his position of comfort lying or sitting in the mother's lap for feeding from the bottle, which they grasp with both the hands. During the feed thereby lessening the possibility of their clutching at the ophthalmoscope with their hands. Darken the room if necessary. Keep the light intensity of the ophthalmoscope down. Do not use mydriatic drops without permission. The doctor should make the child look in the desired direction by making suitable sound or noises with his fingers or with a rattle.

Developmental Stages of Eyes

- Newborn infants dislike light. Turning of head towards light shows discomfort and blinking of eyes.

- At 6 to 8 weeks the infant is alert to moving objects.

- By 12 weeks hand and eye movement may be demonstrated. At this stage lacrimal glands will also respond to emotions.

- At 4 to 5 months of age one inch brick will cause immediate fixation within a distance of one meter.

- Unusual activity continues to improve dramatically from 9 to 12 months and very small objects can be seen and picked up using index finger and thumb.

- At one year of age transverse diameter of cornea is of adult size (12 mm).

- Convergence is well established by 18 months.

- By 4 years visual acuity is 6 x 6.

CHAPTER 12

Examination of the Ear, Nose and Throat

- Examination of Ear
    - External examination
    - Otoscopy
    - Hearing tests
- Examination of Nose
- Examination of Throat

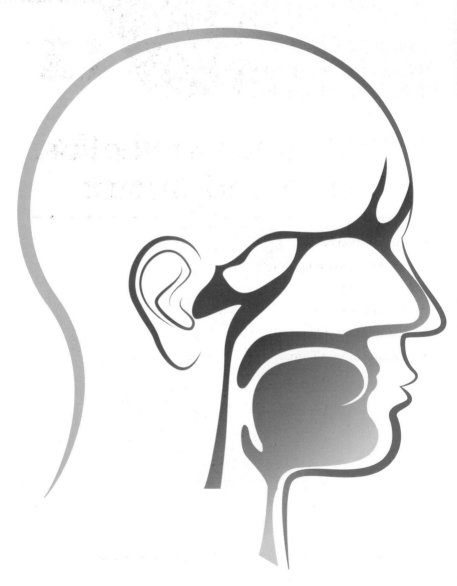

Ear, nose and throat

Examination of the Ear, Nose and Throat

Examination of the Ear

There are three components of ear examination:

1.   External examination
2.   Otoscopy
3.   Assessment of hearing.

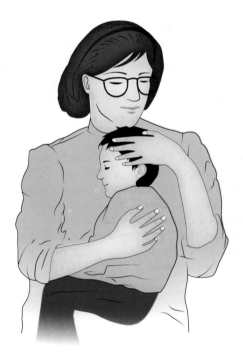

Fig. 12.1   Method of holding child during ear examination

External Examination

Note the shape and the position of the ears. Low set ear is called when the helix (top of the pinna) meets cranium at a level below a horizontal plane from the corner of inner palpebral fissure. It is seen in Treacher-collin syndrome, Down syndrome and various other syndromes, several of which are associated with mental retardation. Abnormalities of the external ear are associated with kidney abnormalities. Pain on pulling the pinna suggests a boil in the external canal.

Otoscopy

The mother should gently but firmly hold the child so that her one hand holds the forehead and other hand around the chest grasps the child's hands. The legs may be held between the mother's thighs (figure 12.1).

To examine the ears of an infant, it is usually necessary to pull pinna downwards and backwards since the canal is directed upward. In older children, the pinna is pulled backward and upward.

Do not push the otoscope in for more than 0.5 cm in infants and 1 cm in older children.

Inspect the canal, one finds a furuncle, (extremely painful) or otitis external in the canal. Also unexpected foreign body may be discovered. Normal ear drum is grayish white and translucent with a clear light deflects. The commonest abnormality deducted is redness which if accompanied by bulging implies with an ear infection. In Glue ear (secretory otitis media) the ear drum is lusterless, dull retracted or bulged with loss of light reflex. Mastoiditis is now very uncommon but when present shows a post auricular swelling or tenderness.

Hearing

The early detection of hearing defect is very important in care of normal babies. If a parent says that the infant is not hearing well, this must be accepted and investigated until disproved. Indications and methods of hearing assessment are described in tables 12.1 and 12.2.

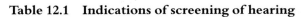

Table 12.1 Indications of screening of hearing

• Low birth weight baby	• Otitis media
• Premature delivery	• Mucopolysaccharoidosis
• Positive family history	• Head injury
• Birth asphyxia	• Torch infection
• Meningitis	• Craniofacial anomaly
• Kernicterous	• Poor school performance
	• Delayed speech

Table 12.2 Methods of screening

• 0–4 months	Startle reflex
• 5–6 months	Localises sound in horizontal plane
• 7–12 months	Localises sound in all planes
• Newborn	Brainstem audiometry
• 6 months-2.5 years	Visual audiometry
• 2.5–5 years	Play audiometry
• Over 5 years	Pure tune audiometry

Examination of the Nose

Note the shape of the nose. A sunken nasal bridge may occur in various disorders like syphilis, down syndrome, hurler syndrome etc. Look for the patency of nose. Air movement through each nostril can be detected by listening with stethoscope or by condensation on a mirror held over the anterior nares. Nasal patency in the newborn can be established by the passing a catheter. In case of choanal atresia, catheter will not pass beyond 5 cms.

141

Check for any discharge from the nose. Running nose or persistent nasal discharge is a common complaint. Clear watery discharge is seen in viral or allergic rhinitis. Purulent discharge suggests sinusitis or adenoidal obstruction. Unilateral serosanguinous nasal discharge is characteristic of a foreign body or nasal diphtheria. Bloody nasal discharge (epistaxis) is common in children. Its common causes are local trauma, nose picking, rhinitis, high grade fever, foreign body and bleeding disorders.

Look for nasal mucosa. Boggy nasal mucosa suggests allergy while nasal polyps suggests cystic fibrosis or allergy.

Reddish mucosa is seen in bacterial infection.

Examination of the Throat

The examination of throat is an important step in the clinical examination of the children. It should be looked into, whatever the illness is for which the child is brought to the doctor.

Infants and children do not like to have their mouth and throat examined, so their examination should be left just for few minutes. You may quickly get a look at the throat as the baby is crying. Allowing the child to play with spatula will help to overcome the fear. Appropriate restrain methods can be used. Infants and children under 4 years can be satisfactorily examined when seated in mother's lap. The tongue depressor should be inserted along the side of the mouth and gum. The alternate method is to lay the baby on his back and restrain with the sheet or by holding the arms. The examiner stands behind the baby and looks into the mouth from above downward. A spoon may be a better substitute for a spatula for infants and children under 4 years.

The older children can be seated or even stand as in case of adults. For adequate inspection of a throat you may require a good source of light, a well-opened mouth and a speedy observer.

Examination of throat and its findings are summarised in Table 12.3

Table 12.3   Examination of Throat

Examination of throat	Findings (Interpretations)
Lips	Angular stomatitis, cheilosis (B-complex deficiency)
Teeth	Caries (poor hygiene)
Gums	Gingivostomatitis (herpes infection) Stippled blue lines (lead poisoning)
Tongue	Pale (anaemia) dry (dehydration) atrophy (iron def, B-12 def, coeliac disease) coated (fungal infection, enteric, scarlet fever)
Buccal mucosa	Koplic spots (measles) aphthous ulcer (crohns diseases)
Palate and Pharynx	Petechiae (thrombocytopenia) vesicles (viral infection) redness (infection)
Tonsils	Red or exudates (infection) enlarged (prone to infection)

'The difference between fiction and reality? Fiction has to make sense.'

Tom Clancy

CHAPTER 13

Examination of the Musculoskeletal System

- Hands and Feet
- Limbs
- Joints and Bones
- Muscles
- Spine and Back

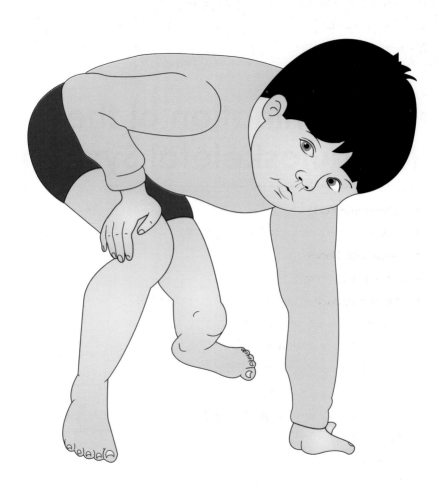

Examination of the Musculoskeletal System

It includes five components of examination:

1. Hands and feet
2. Limbs
3. Bones and joints
4. Muscles
5. Spine and back

Hands and Feet

Note the following abnormalities:

1. Clubbing
2. Curvature of little finger (in mongolism)
3. Deformity of nails
4. Splinter haemorrhage
5. Flat feet (pes cavus) usually up to two years of age.
6. Abnormalities of toes and fingers.

   a. Syndactyly (fusion of digits)

   b. Clinodactyly (incurved digits)

   c. Polydactyly (extra digit)

   d. Arachnodactyly (long thin digit)

7. Abnormalities of feet

   a. Talipes equino varus

   b. Talipes calcanio vulgus

8. Dactylitis, a spindle shaped swelling may occur in tuberculosis, syphilis, rheumatoid arthritis, sarcoidosis, sickle cell anaemia.

Limbs

Look for the following:

1. Deformity, wasting, swelling, paralysis or pseudoparalysis

2. Healthy children tend to be bow legged before the age of 2 years and knock-knees between the age of 2 to 12 years. The limbs, thereafter straighten spontaneously.

3. Increased carrying angle of the elbow as occurs in Turner syndrome

4. Dinner forked deformity of the wrist and hands outstretched may be seen in chorea

5. Flexion deformities involving the finger joints and other joints are seen in disorder like arthrogryposis multiplex congenita.

6. Excessive mobility is seen in Down syndrome

7. There may be amelia (absence of limb), hemilia (absence of distal half of limb), phocomelia (hand or foot attached directly to the trunk). Rarely seen these days, in the past it was due to the use of thalidomide in pregnancy.

8. Upper limbs should be measured from the tip of the acromian to the tip of the middle finger and lower limb from the anterior superior iliac spine to the internal malleolus.

Joints and Bones

1. Palpate bones for any tenderness. Scurvy closely simulates osteitis, so note should be taken of scorbutic rosary or scorbutic changes on X-ray.

2. Joints are tested for a full range of movements. Look for the presence or absence of swelling and local tenderness or pain on active and passive movements to the joints.

3. Dislocation may be evident as gross deformity. Congenital dislocation of the hip is described in the examination of newborn.

4. Arthritis is the inflammation of joints and manifests as:

    a. Redness (rubor).

    b. Pain (dolor).

    c. Heat (colour).

d. Swelling (tumour).

e. Loss of function (functio laesa)

Causes of joint pain are described in table 13.1.

Examination of joints requires knowledge of normal range of movements of a given joint and types of movements at that joint.

Always perform active movement first and then passive movements. Particularly examine the knee, hip and hands.

Table 13.1 Causes of joint pain

Infection	Septic arthritis
	Osteomyelitis lyme disease
	Discitis
	Viral arthritis
	Tuberculosis arthritis
Rheumatological	Rheumatoid arthritis
	Acute rheumatic fever
	Systemic lupus erythematosus
Reactive	Henoch scholein purpura
	Bacilliary dysentry
	Toxic synovitis
Malignant	Leukaemias
	Lymphomas
	Neuroblastoma
	Bone tumours
Hematological	Sickle cell anaemia
	Haemophilia

Skeletal	Trauma
	Slipped capital femoral epiphysis Legg-Calve-Perthes disease
Metabolic	Scurvy

Muscles

(As described in motor system in CNS examination) Gower sign. The child lying on the back on the floor is asked to stand up. He will roll to one side, flex his knee and hips so that he is on all the fours with both knees and both hands on the ground. He then extends his knee and reaches the erect posture by climbing up his own legs, using his hands to get higher up the leg in alternate step. This sign should be checked when suspecting congenital muscular dystrophy.

Spine and Back

This should be routinely examined:

1. Palpate the spinous processes and look for swelling, tenderness and deformity.

2. Undue prominence or gibbus with sharp angulation or lateral displacement of a spinous process usually result from tuberculous destruction of a vertebral body orb mucopolysacroidosis.

3. Rickets can also cause prominence of the spinous processes, but it is an even curvature in the lumbar region, unlike the sharp angulation found in tuberculous disease.

4. Spina bifida can be felt as two separate bony prominences.

5. Neural tube defects can be present and detected usually on inspection. It includes:

   a. Encephalocele-herniation of the brain through congenital skull defects.

   b. Meningocele-open vertebral arches with overlying sac containing CSF.

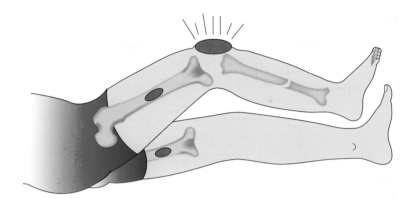

c. Myelomeningocele-Unfused vertebral arches with exposed neural tissue.

d. Spina bifida-failure of fusion of vertebral arches.

e. Anencephaly-congenital absence of the vault.

6. Deformities of spine and back include:

Scoliosis-vertebral column is deformed laterally. It is more evident when the child bends forward to touch his toes or may be suspected if skin creases in the flank area are asymmetrical, Kyphosis-vertebral column has convexity posteriorly Marfan syndrome, Morque's syndrome, Muscle atrophy etc. Lordosis-the vertebral column has convexity anteriorly.

'The reasonable man adapts himself to the world; the unreasonable one persists in trying to adapt the world to himself. Therefore all progress depends on the unreasonable man.'

George Bernand Shaw

'A synonym is a word you use when you can't spell the word you first thought of.'

CHAPTER 14

Examination of the Kidney

- General Examination Related to Kidney
- Abdominal Examination
- Examination of Chest
- Fundoscopy
- Joint Examination
- Ear Examination

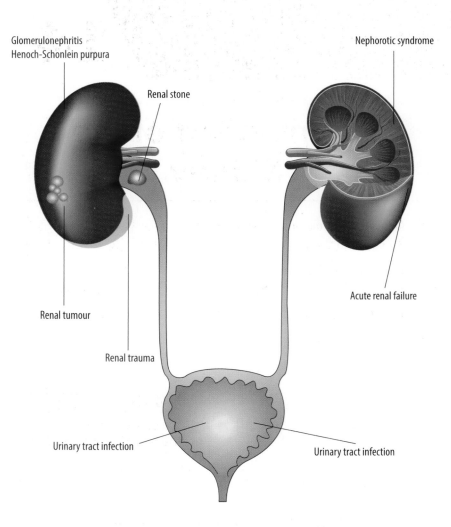

Glomerulonephritis
Henoch-Schonlein purpura

Renal stone

Nephorotic syndrome

Renal tumour

Acute renal failure

Renal trauma

Urinary tract infection

Urinary tract infection

Common renal diseases

Examination of the Kidney

Renal diseases are fairly common in paediatric age group. The presentation is different in different age groups (see table 14.1, 14.2) It is often revealed only by the incidental finding of hypertension or proteinuria especially in older children.

Table 14.1   Conditions in which renal diseases are suspected

Newborn	Post neonatal age
No passage of urine after 24 hours	Passage of blood in urine
	Generalised oedema or ascities
Single umbilical artery	Painful micturation
Flank mass	Backache headache
Family history of renal disease	Decrease urine output
Oligohydramnios	Excessive urine output
Ear abnormalities	Fever without focal symptoms
	Failure to gain weight

Table 14.2   Pains of renal origin

Type of pain	Possible origin
• Constant pain felt in the flank, hypochondrium or iliac fossa	Disease of kidney
• Colicky pain radiating to the groin and in the males, to the testicle	Acute renal obstruction
• Constant backache with pyrexial symptoms	Acute pyelonephritis, renal or perirenal abscess

A child with renal disease, especially when there is chronic renal failure shows a wide variety of clinical features. The examination should proceed by general examination, abdominal examination, of chest and joint examination, followed by possible eye and ear examination.

General Examination Related to Kidney

Following points should be noted while considering renal pathology

General growth:

- Look for signs of growth failure or malnutrition.
- Check skeletal deformity like bowing of leg or knock knee.
- Look for signs of renal rickets.

Skin

- It becomes dry, flanky, pallid, dirty brown in a child with chronic uremia.
- There may be bruises or purpura and scratch marksindicating pruritis.
- Check pitting oedema of ankle, genital swelling and facial puffiness.
- Look for any rashes which may sometime be seen with renal disease like SLE or HSP.
- Don't forget to note pallor.

Check The Blood Pressure

Abdominal Examination

- Look for abdominal distension.
- Palpate both kidney and bladder. The possible causes of palpable kidney are hydronephrosis, polycystic kidney, multicystic kidney, wilms tumour and renal vein thrombosis.
- Note the tenderness of kidney and bladder. It may be due to obstruction or infection.
- Check the shifting dullness and fluid thrill.

Examination of Chest

- Check for the signs of pleural effusion.
- Auscultation is helpful in the diagnosis of pericarditis and pleurisy, by pericardial and pleural rub respectively.

Fundoscopy

- Look for the signs of hypertensive or diabetic retinopathy
- Haemorrhages and exudates may also be seen in vasculitis conditions like systemic lupus erythematosus.

Joint Examination

Examination of the joints are helpful in certain cases because a few of the renal diseases may also involve the joints for example, systemic lupus erythematosis, rheumatoid arthritis, henoch schonlein purpura.

Ear Examination

Sensorineural deafness is seen especially when there is family history of renal disease or hereditary nephritis like alport's syndrome.

> **'Life is a sexually transmitted disease and the mortality rate is one hundred percent.'**
>
> **R.D. Laing**

CHAPTER 15

Examination of the Blood

- Mouth
- Lymph Nodes
- Skin
- Liver and Spleen
- Joint Examination

Blood

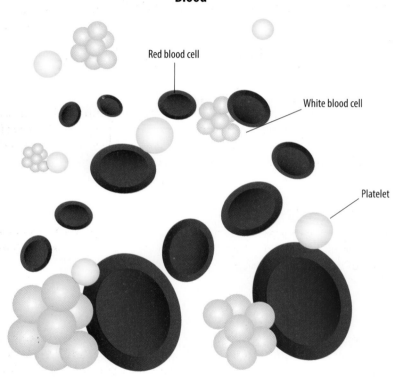

Red blood cell

White blood cell

Platelet

Examination of the Blood

Frequently encountered blood diseases in children are anaemia, bleeding disorder and malignancies like leukaemia and lymphoma. The diagnosis of these disorders begins with the history and physical examination. The causes of anaemia and bleeding disorder are described in table15.1, 15.2, and 15.3, The lymph nodes, liver and spleen are especially important but the skin also gives valuable information about anaemia, infection and bleeding disorders.

Mouth

Mouth should be examined to check angular stomatitis and cheilosis usually seen in iron defeciency anaemia. Red smooth tongue is a feature of folic acid deficiency. Ulceration of mouth may be due to leucopenia and gum bleeding is a familiar feature of thrombocytopenia.

Lymph Nodes

Lymph nodes are enlarged in a variety of blood disorders like lymphoma and leukaemia. It is also a feature of infection and chronic disease.(see chapter of general examination)

Skin

Look for the severity of pallor and any evidence of skin haemorrhage like purpura, ecchymoses or bruises. Bleeding into the skin is the feature of vascular disorder like HSP and thrombocytopenia of any cause.Jaundice may be due to haemolytic anaemia and dusky discolouration is seen in haemosiderosis.

Liver and Spleen

Anaemia and jaundice with an enlarged spleen are features of hemolysis. Liver and spleen may become enlarged in various blood disorder (lymphoma, leukaemia etc). For proper examination see chapter of 'Abdominal examination'

Joint Examination

Joints should be examined when suspecting haemophilia, sickle cell anaemia and HSP.

Table 15.1 Common causes of anaemia

Microcytic anaemia (MCV < 75 fl.)	Normocytic anaemia (MCV 75–100 fl).	Macrocytic anaemia (MCV >100 fl.)
Iron deficiency	Haemolytic anaemia	Megaloblastic (folic acid and B12 deficiency)
Thalassaemias	Haemorrhage	
Lead poisoning	Chronic infection	Bone marrow failure
Pyridoxine def.	Uremia	
Sidroblastic anaemia		
Copper deficiency		

Table 15.2 History related to anaemia

Iron deficiency anaemia	• Age of onset usually 6–24 months
	• History of chronic blood loss
	• Passage of worms
	• Poor dietary intake of iron
	• History of pica
Haemolytic anaemia	• Age of onset(some present at neonatal age and few after 4–6 months usually B cell disorders)
	• Any jaundice
	• History of blood transfusion
	• Family history of anaemia, jaundice, blood transfusion, splenectomy or leg ulcer
Megaloblastic anaemia	• Poor dietary history
	• Chronic diarrhoea
	• Irritability

Table 15.3   Common causes of bleeding disorder

Vascular causes	• Henoch schonlein purpura • Scurvy • Vasculitis syndrome • Malnutrition
Platelet causes	• Idiopathic thrombocytopenic purpura • Drugs • Infections (sepsis and viral infections)
Coagulation disorders	• Congenital (haemophilia, von willibrand disease etc) • Acquired (vitamin K def., liver disease, DIC etc)

Table 15.4   History of a child with bleeding disorder

- Site of bleeding: skin and mucous membrane bleeding is common in vascular and platelet disorders while coagulation disorders commonly presents with deep bleeding or joint bleeding
- Duration and severity of bleeding
- Age of first episode
- Spontaneous or induced by minor or major trauma
- History of bleeding with minor surgical procedure like venipuncture, dental extraction, biopsy or circumcision in male babies
- Any history of drug intake
- Family history of similar illness
- Associated symptoms like joint pain, long standing diarrhoea (vitamin K def.) or stigma of liver disease (jaundice)

Short Cases Examination

General Screening of Genetic Disorder

- About 2% of newborn infants have major anomalies. This incidence is as high up to 5% when malformations detected in childhood are included.

- Almost 50% of the cases are genetic and 40% of the cases are undetected.

- Other causes are chromosomal, environmental or multifactorial inheritance

- Common syndromes to be aware of:

  ○ Trisomy 21 (Down syndrome)

  ○ Trisomy 13 (Patau syndrome)

  ○ Trisomy 18 (Edward syndrome)

  ○ Turner syndrome (45 XO)

  ○ Noonan syndrome (lymphoedema)

  ○ VATER association

  ○ Pierre-Robin sequence

History

- Obtain a three-generational history.

- Always ask about consanguinity.

- Obtain data from both sides of the family.

- Enquire about spontaneous abortions, stillbirths or neonatal death.

- Family history of developmental delay, mental retardation or dysmorphic child.

- Maternal history of drugs and radiation exposure.

Examination

- Look for any dysmorphism or coarse facial features.

- Complete CNS examination.

- Auscultate heart for murmur
- Palpate abdomen for kidneys

Investigations

1. Radiologic examination including views of skull and all long bones. Chest and abdominal films should be obtained when indicated.

2. Ultrasonographic examinations specially of brain and abdomen

3. Cardiac ECHO

4. Computed Tomography (CT) or Magnetic Resonance Imaging (MRI) of brain

5. FISH test and Karyotyping

Evaluation of Heart Disease

History

- Fatigue is the most important symptom of cardiac failure in infant and children.

- A baby in cardiac failure can take only small volumes of milk.

- Shortness of breathing on sucking. The older child tires on walking and breathless.

- Excessive sweating(diaphoresis).

- There may be history of recurrent pneumonia.

- Take a family history of heart disease.

Physical Examination

- General examination:

  ◦ Check for cyanosis, oedema and pallor.

  ◦ Look for failure to thrive and poor growth.

- Signs of heart failure:

  ◦ Tachycardia and tachypnoea

  ◦ Pulmonary crepitations

  ◦ Hepatomegaly

- Pulse and blood pressure:

  ◦ Femoral pulses are weak, delayed or absent in coarctation of the aorta.

  ◦ Blood pressure will be higher in the arms than the legs.

- Precordium:

  ◦ Sternal heave indicates right ventricular hypertrophy (e.g. tetralogy of Fallot, pulmonary hypertension).

  ◦ Murmur: Its grading. type, radiation (back and neck) and examine the child both in sitting and lying position.

Investigations

1. Chest X-ray: for cardiac size and shape, and pulmonary vascularity

2. ECG: for ventricular or atrial hypertrophy

3. Echocardiography: in most of the cases is diagnostic

4. Cardiac catheterisation: when to plan for surgery

Evaluation of Failure to Thrive

History

- Check clinical symptoms: diarrhoea, colic, vomiting, irritability, fatigue or chronic cough.

- Nutritional history: type of feeding (breast fed, formula milk or mixed), time of start of weaning, any feeding problem and present diet.

- Developmental history: either delayed, normal or detoriate

- Past medical history: Low birth weight, prenatal or neonatal problems, recurrent infection or chronic illness.

- Family history: of FTT or genetic disorder. Is there any socio-economic or pschycological issues.

Examination

- General observations.

   ○ Does the child look neglected, ill or malnourished ?

   ○ How does the mother relate to the baby?

   ○ Any dysmorphic features?

- Growth parameters:

   Weight, height and FOC

- Physical examination:

   ○ Look for signs of chronic illness like pallor, murmur, organomegaly.

Investigations

Investigation based on clinical features. Following test should be consider in most of the cases:

1. Complete blood count

2. Serum iron and TIBC

3. LFTs and UCE

4. Urine DR and CS

5. X-ray chest

Specific tests may be needed in some cases when indicated:

1. TB screening (ESR, CXR, MT)

2. Celeac disease test (TTG-IgA)

3. Screening for cystic fibrosis (Delta 508)

Neonatal Jaundice

History

- Age at which jaundice develop? (within 24 hour of birth always requires investigation)
- Is there history of phototherapy or exchange transfusion ?
- Are there any risk factors for infection?
- What is the colour of stool?
- Is there a family history (cystic fibrosis, spherocytosis)?
- Is the baby active, alert and feeding well or lethargic ?
- What is the blood group of mother and father ?

Examination

- What is the extent of the jaundice? (spread from the head to toe)
- Look for pallor.
- Any features of TORCH infection such as petechiae, anaemia or hepatosplenomegaly?
- Is the baby dehydrated? Failure to establish breast-feeding may present with jaundice in the first week of life.
- Is the baby active and alert or are there signs of infection?
- Is there any coarse facial features or umbilical hernia (hypothyroidism)?

Management

- Identify the cause and severity of the jaundice.
- Use phototherapy to bring down the uncongugated bilirubin level.
- In severe haemolytic disease, exchange transfusions may be required to prevent kernicterus.
- Refer to hepatologist if biliary atresia is suspected.
- Check coagulation screen and give vitamin K supplements.

Investigations Needed

- Serum bilirubin

  Total and direct (should be <20%)

- CBC

  Thrombocytopenia suggests viral infection or IUGR

  Anaemia in haemolytic disease

  Neutropenia or neutrophilia in infection

  Blood Group and Coombs test

  ABO and Rhesus incompatibility

- TSH

  For Hypothyroidism

- TORCH screen

  Hepatitis B, cytomegalovirus infection

- LFTs

  Suspecting hepatitis

- Urine metabolic screen:

  Inborn errors of metabolism

- Ultrasound liver

  To visualise biliary tree

- Septic screening

  CBC,CRP,Urine CS, blood CS and cerebrospinal fluid DR

- HIDA scan

  To rule out biliary atresia

  Persistent conjugated hyperbilirubinaemia

- PT and APTT

  Clotting factors are not synthesised well in liver disease, and obstructive jaundice may cause vitamin K deficiency.

  Also deranged in sepsis

Ambiguous Genitalia

HISTORY

Family History

- Parental consanguinity and relatives with ambiguous genitalia, primary amenorrhea, early death, medical issues.
- Autosomal recessive pattern may suggest altered steroidogenesis.
- X-linked recessive pattern may suggest androgen insensitivity syndrome.

Maternal History

- Medications (androgens-progesterones, danazol,testosterone or endocrine disrupters-phenytoin, aminoglutethimide)
- Virilisation before or during pregnancy, prenatal test results

PHYSICAL EXAMINATION

General Examination

- General health
- Dysmorphic features
- Hydration
- Blood pressure

Genital Examination

- Penile/Clitoral length
- Gonads–present/absent, size, location 'Federman's rule–a gonad felt below the inguinal ligament is a testes until proven otherwise'
- Urethral opening–hypospadias, epispadias, virilised urogenital sinus
- Rectal inspection

- Labiosacral fusion–anogenital ratio (distance between anus and posterior fourchette divided by the distance between the anus and the base of the clitoris) of >0.5 suggests Virilisation with some posterior labial fusion.

- External Masculinisation Score–scores scrotal fusion, microphallus, location of urethral meatus and location of each gonad

Initial Laboratory Studies

- Karyotype
- Including FISH with SRY probe
- Serum electrolytes
- Serum 17 alpha hydroxyl progesterone (17–OHP)
- Elevated in most common cause of CAH, 21–hydroxylase deficiency
- Ultrasound of the pelvis/abdomen for mullerian structures
- Serum anti-mullerian hormone (AMH)
- Further testing may be necessary depending on karyotype and other laboratory results. This may include 11–deoxycortisol, cortical, DHEA, ACTH stimulation test, hCG stimulation test.

Asthma-Clinical Findings

GENERAL EXAMINATION

Face: Cushingoid due to steroids (flushed cheeks or moon face), atopy (swollen discoloured eyelids, transverse nasal crease from allergic salute).

Height and Weight

Decreased (not up to the age due to disease or its treatment).

Tanner Staging

Delayed puberty.

Skin

Dry and atopic eczema at elbow or knees.

Nails clubbing due to obliterative bronchiolitis or bronchiectasis.

Pulse

Tachycardia, Pulse paradox

Respiratory rate: Tachypnea at rest, use of accessory muscles.

Hands

Tremors due to beta 2 agonist

CHEST

Inspection

Deformed (increased anteroposterior diameter, Harrison sulcus).

Palpation

Tracheal shift, apex beat shifted, S2 palpable, chest expansion increased.

Percussion

Hyperresonant sound, vocal fremitus increased, vocal resonance increased.

Auscultation

Bilateral wheezing may be found crepts due to overt infection bronchial spasm.

Abdomen: liver and spleen may be palpable due to pushed diaphragm.

Initial Investigations

CBC

IgE-level

X-ray Chest

ABGs

Spirometry

PEFR

Anaemia

HISTORY

1. Severity of Symptoms

- Lethargy, Tachycardia, Pallor, Irritability. Poor intake
- No symptoms commonly seen in chronic anaemia whereas acute anaemia tends to be more symptomatic.

2. Evidence of Hemolysis

a. Changes in urine colour.

b. Jaundice.

c. Haemolytic episodes only in male family members may suggest X-linked disorder (e.g. G6PD deficiency).

3. Prior Therapy or Anemic Episodes

a. Prior anemic episodes, duration, aetiology, and resolution.

b. Prior therapy for anaemia (e.g. failed iron therapy).

4. Blood Loss

a. GI bleeding: changes in stool colour, blood in stools, bowel symptoms.

b. Menstrual losses: duration of periods, flow, and saturation of tampons or pads.

c. Severe epistaxis.

d. If significant blood loss, probe family history for inflammatory bowel disease, polyps, colourectal cancer, hereditary haemorrhagic telangiectasia, von Willebrand disease, platelet disorders, and haemophilia.

5. Underlying Medical Conditions

   a.   Chronic underlying infectious or inflammatory conditions

   b.   Recent illnesses

   c.   Travel to/from areas of endemic infection (e.g. malaria)

6. Prior Drug or Toxin Exposure

   a.   Environmental toxin exposure (e.g. well water containing nitrates)

   b.   Homeopathic or herbal medications

   c.   Risk for lead exposure: housing, paint, cooking materials, poorly glazed ceramic pots

   Pica: eating dirt, paint chips, and any unusual substances (often associated with iron deficiency)

7. Nutritional History

8. Birth History

   Gestational age at birth, Significant loss of blood at birth (may affect the amount of iron stores), History of exchange or intrauterine transfusion, Jaundice or need for phototherapy (may suggest inherited haemolytic anaemia).

9. Growth/Developmental History

   a.   Normal height and weight gain usually eliminate chronic disease as aetiology of anaemia.

   b.   Loss of milestones or developmental delay (in infant with megaloblastic anaemia, may suggest defect of B12 or folate pathways).

10. Family History

   History of anaemias, Splenectomies, Sickle cell disease, G6PD deficiency, cholelithiasis or blood transfusions.

PHYSICAL EXAMINATION

General Examination

1. Evidence of chronic illness or growth failure.

2. Conjunctival pallor, glossitis (associated with B12 and iron deficiency), frontal bossing (seen in Thalassaemia).

3. Lymph adenopathy (leukaemia and lymphomas, chronic diseases, HIV).

4. Skin: petechiae, purpura, jaundice, hemangiomas.

5. Radial anomalies (associated with congenital anaemias, e.g. Fanconi's anaemia).

Cardiovascular System

1. Heart rate

2. Presence of murmur

3. Signs of cardiac failure

Abdominal Examination

1. Hepatomegaly (malignancies, extrameduallary hematopoesis, chronicdiseases).

2. Splenomegaly (haemolytic anaemias, ALL, lymphomas, extrameduallry hematopoesis).

INITIAL LABORATORY STUDIES

1. Complete Blood Count (CBC)

*   Level of Hb to asses the severity of anaemia.

*   Mean corpuscular volume (MCV) to classify micro, normo and macrocytic anaemia.

*   Mentzer index.

*   RPI-Reticulocyte production index (more than 3 indicate haemorrhage or hemolysis).

- Red cell distribution width (RDW): evaluates anisocytosis (normal is 11.5–14.5).

- Leukopenia, Neutropenia, and/or Thrombocytopenia may signify abnormal bone marrow function or increased peripheral destruction of blood cells.

- Reticulocyte count: indication of bone marrow erythropoietic activity.

2. Blood cell smear

    a. RBC size: microcytosis vs macrocytosis

    b. Central pallor: Increased central pallor (iron deficiency and thalassaemia) or no central pallor (spherocytes and reticulocytes).

    c. Fragmented cells (microangiopathic process)

    d. Sickle cells (sickle cell disease)

    e. Elliptocytes (congenital elliptocytosis)

    f. Target cells (thalassaemia, in liver disease, and post-splenectomy).

    g. Bite cells (Heinz body haemolytic anaemia)

3. Special Tests

Some special tests will be helpful when indicated:

    a. Serum iron,ferritin and TIBC

    b. Hb electrophoresis and PCR-DNA for Thalassaemia

    c. Osmotic fragility test

    d. Sickling test

    e. Coombs test-Direct and Indirect

    f. G6PD assay

    g. Bone marrow biopsy

Arthritis

GENERAL INSPECTION

Age

- Under five years (JIA)
- Older age (JAS)

Sex

- Females (JIA)
- Males (JAS)

Skin

- Butterfly malar erythema in SLE.
- Vasculitis rash in SLE.
- Maculopapular rash in systemic JIA.
- Nodules in JIA and JRA.
- Pallor/jaundice or scratch marks in SCD.

UPPER LIMBS

Hands

- Raynaud's phenomenon in SLE.
- Joint swelled or tender in SCD.

Nail

Subungual haemorrhage in SLE.

Palms

- Pallor crease in SCD, JIA
- SLE due to anaemia
- Flexor tenosynovitis in JIA

Elbow

- Epitrochlear nodes in systemic JIA or SLE.
- Rheumatoid nodules in JRA.

Axillae

Lymphadenopathy in SLE and Systemic JIA.

HEAD AND NECK

Hairs

Alopecia (SLE)

Eyes

- Signs of seronegative JIA (iridocyclitis, band keratopathy, glaucoma, changed pupil shape)
- Signs of seropositive JIA (dry eyes, scleritis, episcleritis, scleromalacia performans)
- Cataract in JIA

Mouth

- Ulcers in SLE and SCD.
- Inflamed mucous membrane and petechiae and purpura in SLE.
- Parotid swelling in Sjogrens syndrome

Neck

- Lymphadenopathy in SLE and Systemic JIA
- Laryngeal nodules in JRA. Atlanto-axial sublaxation in JIA

Chest

- Cardiomegaly (SLE, SCD, Systemic JIA)
- Pericarditis (SlE, Systemic JIA)
- Murmur (SCD, SLE)
- Pleural effusion (SLE)
- Pleuritis (Systemic JIA, JIA, SLE and SCD)
- Crepts (SCD)

Abdomen

- Tenderness (SLE, SCD)
- Hepatospleenomegaly (SLE SCD,Systemic JIA)

Lower Limbs

- Hemiplegic or limping in SCD
- Joint swelling or tenderness in SCD

Thalassaemia

The evaluation of thalassaemia begins with a history and physical examination. Physical findings includes the following:

- Typical facial features e.g. prominent checks and teeth
- Growth failure
- Skin colour changes
- Pallor and Jaundice
- Enlarged liver
- Enlarged spleen
- Rapid pulse
- Deformed bones
- Delayed pubertal staging

Tests are necessary to make the diagnosis of thalassaemia. Tests that may be used to evaluate thalassaemia include:

- Check Hb, RBC count, MCV, MCH, Mentzer index, RPI and Retic count.
- Peripheral blood smear
- Haemoglobin electrophoresis and PCR for DNA

Examination of Child with T.O.F

General Inspection

Squatting position (compensatory mechanism)

Restless

Failure to thrive

Growth retardation

Dusky blue skin

Scoliosis (common)

Vitals

Increased temperature (due to infections)

Normal pulse (usually)

Increased respiratory rate

Normal blood pressure (usually)

Face

Pale conjunctivitis (Relative anaemia)

Grey Sclera e engorged blood vessels (including retinal engorgement on fundoscopy)

Cyanosis of Lips (at birth in severe form)

Gingivitis. Bleeding Gums

May be Plethoric (due to polycythemia)

Chest

Left bulging hemi thorax

Apex beat-in 5th ICS medial to mid clavicular line (usually)

Right ventricular pre-dominance on palpation

Left Parasternal Heave-may be noted

Systolic thrill (anteriorly along the left sternal border in 3rd and 4th Parasternal space)

Harsh systolic ejection murmur (over pulmonary area and left sternal border)

Aortic ejection click.

Continuous murmur (in aorto-pulmonary collaterals)

S2 usually single (Pulmonary value closure is not heard)

Soft P2

Peripheries

Cyanosis of nail beds (at birth in severe form)

Clubbing of fingers and toes (after 3–4 months). Tender joints (Arthritis due to hypoxic arthropathy)

PAROXYSMAL HYPER CYANOTIC ATTACKS

(Blue or TET Spells in 1st two years of life)

- Restless
- Hyperpneic
- Increased cyanosis
- Gasping respiration
- Syncope
- Convulsions
- Hemiparesis in severe form
- Unconsciousness

Cardiac Murmur

History

1. Growth failure, Poor weight gain/FTT

2. History of cyanotic or apneic spell

3. In infants-feeding difficulties, tachypnea, irritability, sweating

4. Older children-exercise intolerance, syncope, chest pain

5. History of recurrent Pneumonia

6. Birth history-prenatal conditions, exposure to drugs in pregnancy

7. Family history of cardiac lesions or other anomalies physical exam.

General Examination

1. Growth failure

2. Cyanosis/ digital clubbing

3. Oedema

4. Presence of non-cardiac malformations. Incidence of congenital heart disease increase with other anomalies

Cardiovascular System

1. Pulses-rate, rhythm, volume, character, comparison and delay

2. BP and difference in upper and lower extremities

3. Jugular venous pressure

4. Active or hyper dynamic precordium

5. Signs of CHF-tachypnea, liver enlargement, rales, periorbital oedema.

6. Signs of increased pulmonary pressure-Loud S2, systolic murmur, cyonosis.

7. Murmur-intensity, location, timing, does it change with position and with respiration,

8. Heart Sound-First and Second heart sound-intensity, splitting of 2nd heart sound. Usually with increased pulmonary pressure, the 2nd sound will become louder and single.

9. Additional Sounds-Gallop, clicks, snaps etc

Functional Murmurs

1. Venous hums-usually continuous and disappear in supine position. Heard best under clavicles. Due to turbulence in the jugular venous system.

2. Carotid bruits-base of the neck.

3. Pulmonary flow-ULSB. Due to turbulence from the pulmonary artery ejection

4. Vibratory-LLSB-high pitched and less than grade 2. Doesn't radiate. Changes with position of the child. Intensity will increase with exercise, fever, and excitement.(all associated with increased HR).

Findings in the Child with Rickets

General Inspection

- Failure to thrive

- Listlessness

- Short stature (adult of less than 5 feet tall) {chronic renal disease, malabsorption rickets}.

- Weight loss (decreased intake or malabsorption rickets)

- Strider (laryngeal spasm)

- Proximal muscle weakness (rickety myopathy or 'floppy baby syndrome' or 'slinky baby')

- Uncontrolled Muscle cramps all over body. (Hypocalcemiatetany).

- Fits (hypocalcemic seizures)

- Fractures

Head

- Asymmetrical or odd-shaped skull (craniosynostosis)

- Craniotabes (soft skull) { also in osteogenesis imperfect, hydrocephalus and syphilis}

- Delayed fontanel closure

- Alopecia (vitamin D-dependent rickets type 2)

Face

- Frontal bossing

- Anaemia (chronic renal failure).

- Dental problems (-delayed formation of teeth
  - Defects in the structures of teeth
  - Holes in enamel
  - Dental caries)

Chest

- Costochondral junctions widening (rachitic rosary or rickety rosary)
- Harrison groove (during inspiration)
- Intercostal and subcostal recession (respiratory infection and atelectasis---in vitamin D deficiency disorder)

Back

- Scoliosis
- Kyphosis
- Lordosis

Abdomen

- Protruded abdomen
- Lax skin (malabsorption)
- Hepatosplenomegaly (anemic failure)

Hands

- Double malleoli sign (due to metaphyseal hyperplasia)
- Widening of wrist
- Bone and joint tenderness

Legs

- Toddlers: bowed legs (genu varum)
- Older children:-knock-knees (genu valgum)

  Windswept deformity (combination of valgus deformity of 1 leg and varus deformity of the other leg)
- Anterior bowing of tibia and femur
- Coxa vara (deformity of hip)
- Leg pain

Gait

- Waddling gait (due to weakness of proximal muscles of pelvic girdle)
- Delayed walking

Nephrotic Syndrome

Physical Findings in Someone with Nephrotic Syndrome May Include

- Puffiness of face.
- Generalised swelling.
- Swelling all over the body.
- Leg swelling.
- High blood pressure.

Physical Findings in Someone with Kidney Failure Include

- Pale skin.
- Facial swelling.
- Leg swelling (bilateral)
- Foot swelling (bilateral)
- Arm swelling (bilateral)
- Abdominal swelling
- Scrotal swelling
- Excessive bruising
- Muscle weakness
- Weight gain
- Confusion

Tests That May be Used to Evaluate Nephrotic Syndrome Include

- 24-hour urine for creatinine clearance and total protein
- Complete blood count

- UCE.
- Serum albumin levels: usually less than 2.5 gm/dl
- Total serum protein.
- Urine analysis.

  Usually contains excessive protein
- 24-hour urine protein: may show over 2.5 grams of protein Additional tests that may be used to evaluate the kidneys include:
- Ultrasound KUB
- Intravenous pyelogram
- Kidney biopsy
- Renal arteriogram

Acute Glomerulonephritis

Physical Findings in Those with Acute Glomerulonephritis May Include

- Confusion
- Lethargy
- Excessive sleepiness
- Pale and Dry skin.
- Leg swelling
- Foot swelling (bilateral)
- Facial swelling, Worse around the eyes
- Enlargement of the liver
- High blood pressure

Tests that may be Used to Evaluate Acute Glomerulonephritis Include

- Serum calcium level
- Serum phosphate level
- Complete blood count
- Urinalysis
- 24-hour urine for creatinine clearance

Additional Tests that May be Used to Evaluate the Kidneys Include

- Ultrasound-KUB
- Abdominal CT scan
- Intravenous pyelogram
- Kidney biopsy
- MRI scan of the abdomen
- Renal arteriogram
- Kidney biopsy

Examination of an Unconscious Child

General Inspection

- Unconscious/unresponsive
- Decorticate or Decerebrate postures

Any Cranial Trauma

- Raccoon eyes
- Bleeding from nose or ears
- Neck splint and collar

Specific Breathing Odour

(of alcohol, uremia, diabetic ketoacidosis, hepatic coma)

Breathing Patterns

- Deep, rapid respiration (acidosis)
- Cheyne-Stokes breathing (periodic)
- Kussmaul's breathing
- Central point hyperventilation
- Deep gasping respiration with hiccoughs (ataxic respiration)

Any Obvious Fracture or Traction Applied. Assess Level of Consciousness (G.C.S.) Vitals

- Hypo or hyperthermia (sepsis, Pneumonia, meningitis, brain abscess)
- May be no pulse palpable (circulatory Failure-search for external and internal. haemorrhage–if trauma suspected)
- May be normal, increased or gasping respiration
- May be increased or decreased blood pressure

Head and Neck

- Scalp Oedema/Haematoma/ Fracture

- Battle sign :(Bruising of skin behind pinna-indicator of middle cranial fossa fracture)

- Bleeding from nose or ears

- Splint around neck (Fracture of cervical spine)

- Neck stiffness (meningeal irritation -if no injury)

Face and Eyes

- Unequal Pupillary size

- Larger-Occulomotor Palsy

- Smaller-Horner's syndrome

- Pupillary reaction to light:

- Pinpoint pupil, not reacting to light(pontine haemorrhage.thallamic haemorrhage)

- Pinpoint pupil, reacting to light(opium Poisoning).

- Pupil dilated and reacting to light(systemic atropine administration).

- Dilated and fixed Pupil (cerebral herniation,severe brain injury impending death).

- Sign of III, IV or VI nerve palsy

- Doll's Eye movement (Positive in comatose patient when brainstem is intact)

- Nystagmus (not in comatose patient)

- Spontaneous Ocular movement (infection or lesion in posterior cranial fossa)

- Pale conjunctive (anemic Failure)

- Jaundice (hepatic /uremic coma)

- Cyanosis of lips (respiratory Failure)

- Rashes, Petechiae

- Occulcovestibular, corneal, cough and gag reflexes
- Otoscopy
- Bleeding from external Auditory meatus
- Haemotympanum (blood behind eardrum)

Chest

- Indrawing (suprasternal, subcostal or intercostals)
- Spider nevi
- Any Murmur on CVS examination
- Any positive finding on respiratory examination (like dull percussion note, fine crepts, wheezes etc)

Abdomen

- Distended abdomen
- Umbilical hernia
- Prominent vessel
- Decreased liver span (may be)
- Splenomegaly
- Fluid thrill

Peripheries

- No peripheral pulses palpable (circulatory failure)
- Pitting oedema
- Bruises
- Peripheral cyanosis
- Clubbing
- Pallor palmar creases (anemic failure)
- Liver palms (hepatic coma)

CNS

- Level of consciousness.
- Sign of cranial nerve palsy.
- Abnormal flaccidity (hemiplegic).
- Focal neurological Signs.
- Plantar reflex-extensor (mostly).
- Tendon reflexes-Asymmetrical.
- Sign of meningeal irritation.
- Fundoscopy.
- Papilloedema (raised Intracranial Pressure).
- Retinal haemorrhages or exudates.
- Intra-arterial emboli.

Clinical Findings of a Child with Down Syndrome

General Inspection

- Short stature
- Obese (sometimes normal)
- Weight and head circumference is less than usual
- Hypotonic
- Fits

Head

- Brachycephaly with flat occiput
- Fontanel wide open
- Mild microcephaly

Face

- Flat face
- Upward slanted palpebral fissures
- Epicanthal folds
- Speckled irises (brushfield spots)
- Nystagmus
- Strabismus
- Cataract
- Small nose
- Flat nasal bridge
- Small dysplastic ears
- Open mouth
- Protruding tongue
- Small teeth
- Short hard palate
- Seborrhea
- Xerosis

Neck and chest

- Poor moro's reflex
- Short neck
- Atlantoaxial instability
- Redundant skin
- Short sternum
- Murmur (of VSD, ASD, or PDA)

Abdomen

- Palpable mass (may be due to duodenal atresia)
- Umbilical hernia
- Cutis marmorata

Hands

- Shortened metacarpals and phalanges
- Short fifth digit with clinodactyly
- Single transverse palmer crease
- Recurrent joint dislocations (shoulder, elbow, thumb)
- Joint hyperflexibility

Pelvis and Lower Extremities

- Pelvic dysplasia
- Recurrent dislocation of knee joint
- Wide gap between first and second toes

Genitalia and Anus

- Smaller genitalia.
- Imperforate anus.

Skin Examination

History

Following points will be noted while taking history related to skin lesion:

1. Age of onset

2. Progression of symptom

3. Associated symptom (pain, pruritus)

4. Associated systemic features (fever, malaise, pain, weight loss) provide important clues to the history

5. Other important questions include history regarding allergies, environmental exposure, family history, drug history and past history of similar episode

Physical Examination

Examination of skin includes systemic examination of the entire body, along with examination of the mucous membranes, nails, hair, teeth (all of ectodermal origin) are also involved in the examination. In the presence of skin lesion following points should be noted,

1. Symmetrical or asymmetrical

2. Centrifugal or centripetal

3. Flexor or extensor bias

4. Localised or generalised

5. Exposed areas or covered areas

6. Irritation or scaling

7. Involvement of mucous membrane (eye, mouth, nose, anus etc.)

Common Manifestations of Skin Lesion

PRIMARY SKIN LESION

Macule

Flat, well circumscribed<1 cm in diameter distinguished from surrounding skin by colour only with variable size and shape, which may be erythematous, pigmented or purpuric.

Papule

Elevated, circumscribed solid lesion <1 cm in diameter, which may be scaly or ulcerated or may become pustular.

Plague

Similar to papule but >1 cm in diameter.

Nodule

Large, palpable papule that extends 2 cm deep into the dermis or subcutaneous tissue.

Tumour

Similar to nodule, but extends >2 cm into the dermis or subcutaneous tissue.

Vesicle

Small fluid filled (usually clear or straw coloured) epidermal lesion, 1 cm in diameter.

Bulla

Similar to vesicle, but>1 cm in diameter, which may be flaccid or tense, reflecting Depth within the skin.

Purpura

Macule resulting from extravasated blood into the skin, does not blanch with pressure.

Petechia

Small red to purple circumscribed macule resulting from extavasated blood, measuring a few millimeters in diameter.

Ecchymosis

Larger. haemorrhagic patch or plaque resulting from extravasated blood.

Pustule

Papule that contains purulent exudates which may have initial papular base often Surrounded by erythema.

Wheal

Transient, rounded or flat topped oedematous plague, varies greatly in size and may have an annular or gyrate configuration.

Cyst

Papule or nodule with an epidermal lining composed of fluid or solid material.

SECONDARY SKIN LESION

Scale	Results from abnormal keratinization, may be fine or sheet like.
Crust	Dried collection of serum and cellular debris.
Erosion	Moist, shallow epidermal depression with loss of superficial epidermis.
Ulcer	Circumscribed, depressed, focal loss of entire epidermis into the dermis Heals with scarring.
Atrophy	Shallow depression that results from thinning of epidermis or dermis.
Scar	Thickened, firm and discoloured collection of connective tissue that Result from dermal damage initially pink but lightens with time.
Sclerosis	Circumscribed or diffuse hardening of skin usually forms in a plague.
Lichenification	Accentuated skin lesions /markings that result from thickening of the epidermis.
Excoriation	Superficial linear erosion that is caused by scratching.
Fissure	Linear break within the skin surface that usually is painful.

Initial Diagnostic Evaluation and Screening Tests

A detailed history and thorough examination is usually sufficient because lesions most of the times are visible.Diagnostic tests are used only for few occasion and most of the times required for the confirmation of the diagnosis Initial test include KOH for fungi and dermatophytes and gram staining for bacterial infections. The diagnostic test for dermatological purpose is skin biopsy, which is required for only few occasions. Specimen is taken through punch biopsy which is very simple and painless procedure.

Inborn Errors of Metabolism

Findings Suggestive of an Acute Inborn Error of Metabolism Often Confused with Sepsis.

1. Poor feeding
2. Persistent vomiting
3. Lethargy
4. Convulsions resistant to IV glucose or calcium
5. Hypotonic or spasticity
6. Tachypnea/Kussmaul breathing/apnea
7. Failure to thrive
8. Coma
9. Not responding to conventional therapy

Findings Suggestive of a Chronic IEM Course.

1. Developmental delay (especially regression).
2. Unexplained Jaundice
3. Seizures resistant to anticonvulsant therapy
4. Movement disorder
5. Peripheral muscle weakness
6. Cardiomyopathy
7. Hepatosplenomegaly
8. Resistant Hypoglycemia
9. Renal failure
10. Cataracts
11. Retinal abnormalities
12. Macrocephaly
13. Dysmorphic features
14. Unusual body odour

Initial Investigations

1. CBC, differential, and platelets
2. Serum electrolytes
3. Arterial blood gas
4. Serum glucose
5. Plasma ammonia level
6. Urine for reducing substances, ketones and organic acids
7. Amino acids chromatograph
8. Liver function tests if the child has encephalopathy

Clinical Findings in the Child with Hypothyroidism

General Inspection

- Lethargic
- Hypotonic
- Birth weight and length normal
- Increase weight with advancing age due to water retention
- Stunted growth with age
- Short extremities
- General pallor with sallow complexion
- Carotinemia (yellow discolouration of skin but sclera remain normal)
- Skin dry and scaly
- Hoarse voice

Head

- Head size normal or slightly increased
- Anterior and posterior fontanelle are widely open
- Scalp is thickened
- Hairs are coarse, brittle and scanty
- Hairline far down on the forehead

Face

- Loss of lateral aspects of eyebrows
- Eyes appear far apart
- Palpebral fissures are narrow
- Swelling of the eyelids
- Bridge of the broad nose is depressed
- Mouth is open
- Protruded thick broad tongue
- Dentition delayed

Neck and Chest

- Neck short and thick
- Deposits of fat above the clavicle and between neck and shoulder
- Bradycardia
- Apex beat away from the mid-clavicular line in 5th intercostal space
- Heart murmurs

Abdomen

- Abdomen large
- Umbilical hernia

Extremities

- Slow pulse
- Hands are broad
- Fingers are short
- Non-pitting oedema in lower extremities
- Muscle pseudohypertrophy particularly in calf muscle (Kocher-Debre-Semelaigne syndrome)
- Slow relaxation phase of reflexes

Genitals

Swollen genitals

Myxoedema Coma

- Altered level of consciousness.
- Nasal flaring
- Intercostal and subcostal recessions
- Generalised oedema

Hepatomegaly

Liver edge 3.5 cms. below the right costal margin in newborns and 2 cms below the RCM in older children. The average liver span is 4–5 cms in newborns and 6– 8 cms in children at 12 years of age.

History

- Jaundice or History of contact with jaundice patient
- Family History of liver disease
- Family history of metabolic disease, neurodegenerative disease
- Developmental delay may indicate CNS storage disease Maternal infections during the pregnancy (TORCH)
- Umbilical catheter use in the newborn period
- Risk factors for Viral hepatitis e.g blood transfusion history of drug intake

General Examination

- Dysmorphic features? mucopolysaccharidoses
- Fever systemic disease or infection
- Jaundice
- Oedema
- Increase of lymph nodes-Infection or neoplasia
- Palmer erythemia
- Hemangiomas

Abdominal Examination

- Splenomegaly-portal hypertension, infiltration by malignancies and storage diseases, haemolytic disease, haemoglobinopathies.
- Prominent veins
- Ascites

Eye-cataracts. Keyser Fleischer rings, chorioretinitis, developmental delay and neurologic deterioration-characteristic of storage diseases and wilson's disease.

Laboratory Evaluation

- CBC and diff, platelet count, reticulocyte counts, and smear
- Liver function test

Indication of liver cell destruction. Alanine aminotransferase is more specific than aspartate aminotransferase for liver pathology

- PT, APTT and Albumin are markers for liver synthetic function
- Bilirubin-evidence of obstruction, cell damage, and hemolysis
- Alkaline phosphatase and gamma glutamyl transpeptidase indicate biliary obstruction
- Serum glucose
- Viral studies for Hepatitis A, B, and C

Imagingÿ

- Ultrasound-define size, consistency, small masses, and blood flow.
- CT and MRI
- Biopsy-will demonstrate parenchymal changes, presence of storage materials, and tissue for enzyme identification

Clinical Findings of Nutritional Syndrome

MARASMUS

General Inspection

- Irritable on handling, alert followed by listlessness
- Loose and wrinkled skin
- Muscle wasting particularly of buttocks and thighs
- Growth retardation
- Hypotonic
- Pallor
- Oedema never present
- Skin and hair changes are absent

Vitals

- Hypothermia
- Bradycardia
- Hypotension

Face

- Simian facies---face is shrunken and wizened (due to loss of buccal pad of fat)
- Chest
- Prominent rib cage

Abdomen

Protuberant abdomen (due to hypotonic muscles) with intestinal pattern visible.

Extremities

- Tendon reflexes are diminished.
- Plantar reflexes may be absent in extreme cases.

KWASHIORKOR

General Inspection

- Lethargic, apathetic, and/or irritable
- Growth retardation
- Loss of muscle tissue but some subcutaneous fat
- Generalised oedema
- Pallor
- 'Flaky paint dermatitis' in covered areas with darkening of skin in irritated areas
- Depigmentation occurs after desquamation of these areas
- Flag sign (alternating bands of light and normal colours)
- Shiny and edematous skin.
- Erosions.
- Poor wound healing, petechiae

Vitals

- Hypothermia
- Bradycardia
- Hypotension

Head and Face

- Moon face
- Dull, sparse, brittle hair

- Alopecia.
- Broomstick eyelashes

Abdomen

- Distended abdomen
- Hepatomegaly
- Ascites

Extremities

- Pitting oedema (including periorbital oedema)
- Loss of knee and ankle reflexes

Signs of Micronutrient Deficiency

Eyes

- Dry eyes
- Pale conjunctiva
- Bitot spots (vitamin A)

Mouth

- Angular stomatitis
- Cheilitis
- Glossitis
- Spongy bleeding gums (vitamin C)
- Parotid enlargement
- Chvostek sign (hypocalcemia)

Teeth

- Enamel mottling
- Delayed eruption

Extremities

- Trousseau sign (hypocalcemia)
- Skeletal deformity (due to calcium, vitamin D, or vitamin C deficiencies)
- Koilonychia, thin and soft nail plates, fissures or ridges

Hearing Loss

The deaf are those in whom the sense of hearing is non-functional for ordinary purposes of life.'

The Degree of Hearing Loss

The degree of hearing loss varies from:

- Mild   (20–30 dB)
- Moderate   (30–50 dB)
- Severe   (50–70 dB)
- Profound   (> 70 dB)

The Types of Hearing Loss

Hearing loss is divided mainly into; peripheral type of loss and central type of loss:

The peripheral type is further divided into; conductive, sensorineural or mixed. The disease processes and interferes with the sound conduction to reach cochlea results in conductive hearing loss. It is the most common type in children.

Causes of CHL can be congenital or acquired. Congenital causes include meatal atresia or stenosis, fixation of stapes foot plate, fixation of malleus head, ossicular discontinuity and congenital cholesteatoma. Acquired causes include obstruction of external ear by impactions of cerumen, foreign body, or furuncle. In the middle ear, perforations of TM, acute or serous otitis media, disruption or fixation of ossicles, blockage of eustachian tube can cause CHL. Hearing loss resulting from lesions of the cochlea, VIIIth nerve or central auditory pathways is known as sensorineural hearing loss.

It can also result from congenital or acquired causes. Any anomaly of the inner ear by prenatal or perinatal factors can cause congenital SNHL. Acquired causes include disease,ototoxic drugs(aminoglycosides, loop diuretics and chemotherapeutic agent) noise induced hearing loss, trauma to the VIIIth nerve or perilymphatic fistula of the round or oval window membrane. Temperal bone fractures trauma to labyrinth, systemic disorders can also cause SNHL. A combination of CHL and SNHL is known as mixed hearing loss.

AETIOLOGY

Infection Causes

Prenatal factors causing congenital SNHL include CMV, toxoplasmosis and syphilis in which CMV is the most common organism and HSV is rare, while the Rubella infection is very uncommon now due to its effective vaccination programs. Prenatal screening is very important as any of these organisms can cause hearing loss. Other organisms which can cause hearing loss postnatally include strep. Pneumoniae, haemophilus influenza type b, parvovirus, lyme disease, varicella, mumps and rubella but they are very uncommon due to the effective vaccinations programs.

Genetic Causes

Autosomal dominant causes are responsible for 10% of SHNL, in which the waard enburg type I, type II and branchio-otorenal syndromes are the most common. Autosomal recessive causes are probably responsible for 80% of SHNL. The most common syndromes include in autosomal recessive SNHL are Usher syndrome, Pendred syndrome and the jervell and long large Nielsen syndrome. Alsteom syndrome and isolter syndrome are the less common conditions of SNHL. Many conditions express themselves soon after birth while many conditions manifest late. Some children are symptomatic in which making of diagnosis is not difficult, but in many cases, children may be asymptomatic. Norric disease, Alport syndrome, Nance deafness and otopalatal digital syndrome are the sex linked causes associated with SNHL. Turner syndrome can result in CHL, SNHL or mixed hearing loss.

Physical Causes

It include agenesis or malformation of cochlear structure and anomalies of semicircular canal. These anomalies can be associated with prenatal infection. These anomalies probably occur before the 8th week of gestation.

Hearing loss can also be associated with Pierre Robin, Teacher Collins, Klippel-Feil, crouzon and bronchio-otorenal syndromes.

Hearing Impairment Effects

Impairment of hearing may vary from mild to severe or profound. It may be unilateral or bilateral. It may be conductive, sensorineural or mixed, when there is little or no hearing, the term deafness is used. The nature and degree of hearing loss also vary from person to person. Hearing loss can affect adversely speech, social, emotional or behaviour development of a child.

Audiometric Tests

Pure Tone Audiometry

It is done by audiometer, an electronic device which provides pulse tones, assessment of hearing is done independently for each ear by the use of earphones. Tuning fork tests can also be used for assessment of hearing. When tuning fork is used, vibrations are transmitted by the skull bones as sound energy to the inner ear. In a normal ear or in children with hearing loss of sensorineural type, thresholds of the air and bone conduction are same. The difference in the thresholds of air and bone conductions is called air bone gap (A-B gap) and it is a measure of the degree of conductive deafness.

Speech Audiometry

In this test, measurement of patient's ability to hear and to understand speech is done.

Speech Reception Threshold

In this test, 50% of the words are repeated correctly by the patient. A set of spondee words (two syllable words with equal stress on each syllable) e.g. sunlight, daydream etc is delivered through the headphone of an audiometer to each ear. An average of pulse tone threshold of three speech frequencies (500, 1000, 2000 Hz) are used in SRT. Pictures can be used for those who cannot repeat words clearly for the SRT.

Play Audiometry

It is used for the children between the ages of 30 months to 5 years. Usually activities such as placing rings on a peg, dropping blocks in a bucket or completing a puzzle are responses in play audiometry.

Visual Reinforcement Audiometry

For children 6 months to 30 months, VRA is used. Toy reinforces is used in this technique and the head turning response of the child is observed.

Behavioural Observation Audiometry

It is used for the infants less than 5 months of age. In this technique, observations of an infant are done by reflexive responses to complex test sounds.

Auditory Brainstem Responses

It is a non-invasive technique used to elicit brainstem responses to auditory stimulations by clicks or tone bursts. It measures hearing sensitivity in the ear with 1000–4000 Hz. It is used as screening procedure to determine the threshold of hearing in infants, and in children who do not cooperate and in malingerers. It is also used to diagnose retrocochlear or brainstem pathology. In a normal person, 5–7 waves are produced. The I, II and V waves are most stable and are used in measurements. The waves are studied for absolute latency, interwave latency and the amplitude.

Tympanometry

It provides a graph of the ability of the middle ear to transmit sound energy (admittance or compliance) or impede sound energy. Equipment consists of probe which fits into the external auditory canal. Admittance is expressed in unit called a millimho (mmh) or as a volume of air (ml). When a tympanic membrane is struck by a sound, its energy is absorbed and the other is reflected. An immobile TM would reflect more of sound energy than a non-mobile one.

Acoustic Reflex

This test is useful to assess hearing in infants and in young children, to detect cochlear pathology, to detect VII and VIIIth cranial nerve lesions and the lesion of brainstem. In patients with conductive hearing loss, these reflexes are usually absent due to the abnormality of the transfer system and this test is based on a fact that a loud sound, above the threshold of hearing of a particular ear, causes bilateral contraction of the stapedial muscles which can be detected by tympanometry.

Otoacoustic Emissions: (OAEs)

OAEs sounds are produced by outer hair cells of a normal cochlea and they are low intensity sounds detected by sensitive amplifying processes. These sounds are present when outer hair cells are healthy, and absent when they are damaged. These sounds travel from the cochlea (outer hair cells) to the ear canal by passing basilar membrane, perilymph, oval window, ossicles and tympanic membrane. OAEs are divided into two types: Spontaneous OAEs which are present in normal hearing persons where hearing loss does not exceed 30 dB. ransient evoked OAEs are used to check the cochlea integrity. OAEs are used as a screening test of hearing in neonates and uncooperative children. They are also used to diagnose retrocochlear pathology and to distinguish between cochlea and retrocochlear hearing loss.

CHAPTER 17

Outlines of Electrocardiography

- Indications
- Mathematics
- Sequence of Reading
- Rate
- Rhythm
- P-Wave
- P-R Interval
- QRS Complex
- Q-T Inetrval, S-T Segment and T-Wave
- VentricularHypertrophy
- Criteria of Bundle Branch Block
- Axis Deviation
- Classification of Congenital Heart Disease based on ECG

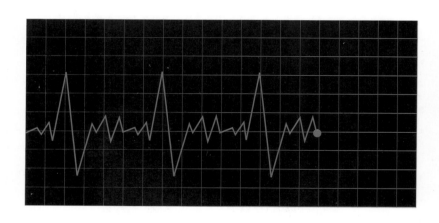

Outlines of Electrocardiography

Indications

- Cardiac arrhythmias or conduction defects
- Congenital heart disease
- Electrolyte imbalance
- Rheumatic fever
- Myocardial disease
- Pericardial disease

Mathematics

- Paper speed 25 mm/second
- Large square 0.2 second and 5 mm
- Small square 0.04 second and 1 mm
- Vertical height of large square 1 mm

Sequence of Reading

- Rate and rhythm
- P-wave and P-R interval
- QRS complex
- Q-T and S-T segments
- T-wave
- Ventricular hypertrophy
- Bundle branch block
- Axis deviation

Rate

Count number of bold lines between two R waves, if it is immediate to next line then rate will be 300/minute with subsequent lines it will be 150, 100, 75, 60, and 50. Causes of increased and decreased heart rate are described in table 16.1.

Rhythm

Regular rhythm is demonstrated by equal interval between two waves specially R-waves. If irregular then check either regularly irregular or irregularly irregular.

P-wave

Best checked in lead II and V. Note the following abnormalities.

- Bifid/inverted/broader than 2.5 mm indicates left atrial hypertrophy (P-mitrale)

- Height greater than 2.5 mm indicates right atrial hypertrophy (p-pulmonale)

P-R interval

Normal values of P-R interval in different age groups are described in table 16.2.

It is best seen in lead II and V. It is prolonged in Ebstein anomaly, rheumatic heart disease, hyperkalemia, myocarditis, endocardial cushion defect. Short P-R interval is seen in wolff parkinson white syndrome. It is variable in 2nd degree heart block.

QRS Complex

Normal values in different age groups and abnormalities are described in table 16.3.

Q-T interval, S-T segment and T-wave (Table 16.3, 16.4)

Ventricular Hypertrophy

Left Ventricular Hypertrophy

Following are the parameters for left ventricular hypertrophy.

1. The sum of height squares of S-wave and R-wave in lead V is > than 35 sqs.

2. Left axis deviation

3. Ventricular activation time greater than 0.04 second. (breadth of R-wave)

Right Ventricular Hypertrophy

1. The sum of height squares of R-wave and S-wave in lead V is > 35 sqs.

2. Right axis deviation

Criteria of Bundle Branch Block

Right Bundle Branch Block

1. Right axis deviation

2. Prolong QRS complex

3. S-T depression

4. T-wave inversion

Left Bundle Branch Block

1. Left axis deviation

2. Prolong QRS complex

3. S-T depression

4. T-wave inversion

Axis Deviation

Check QRS wave (either positive or negative) in a VF and lead I and decide as described in Table 16.6. Causes of axis deviation are described in Table 16.5

Table 16.1 Causes of increased and decreased heart rate (sinus rhythm)

Sinus Bradycardia	Sinus Tachycardia
• Sleep	• Anxiety
• Jaundice	• Fever
• Beta blockers	• Anaemia
• Athletes	• Sympathomimetic drugs
• Raised intracranial pressure	• Hyperthyroidism
• Hypothyroidism	

Table 16.2 Normal values of PR, QT and ST intervals

P-R Interval	QT Interval
• 0.08 second (0–3 years)	0.4 second
• 0.10 second (3–16 years)	**ST Interval**
• 0.12 second (> 16 years)	0.32 second

Table 16.3 Abnormal QRS complex and QT interval

Increased QT Interval	Wide QRS
• Hypocalcemia	• Bundle branch block
• Myocarditis (viral or rheumatic)	• WPW syndrome
• Quinine	• Ventricular arrhythmia
• Hypokalemia	• Hyperkalemia
Decreased QT Interval	• Quinidine toxicity
• Hypercalcemia	
• Digitalis effect	

Table 16.4   ST segment and T-wave abnormalities

ST Depression/ T-Wave Inversion	ST Elevation
• Myocarditis	• Hyperkalemia
• Digitalis toxicity	• Pericarditis
• Hypokalemia	**Peak T-Wave**
• Normal newborn	• Hyperkalemia
	• Posterior infarct
	• Left ventricular hypertrophy

Table 16.5   Causes of axis deviation

Right Axis Deviation	Left Axis Deviation
• Right ventricular hypertrophy	• Left ventricular hypertrophy
• Atrial septal defect	• Atrioventricular septal defect
	• Tricuspid atresia

Table16.6   Axis deviation (note QRS. complex)

Normal axis	Right axis
• +ve aVF	• +ve aVF
• +ve lead I	• -ve lead I
Left axis:	**Extreme right axis:**
• -ve aVF	• -ve aVF
• +ve lead I	• -ve lead I

Table 16.7   Specific ECG findings

Hyperkalemia	Hypokalemia	Wolf Parkinson White Syndrome
• Prolonged P-R interval • Wide QRS complex • Peaked T-wave • No P wave • ST elevation	• ST depression • T-wave inversion • Appearance of u-wave	• Short P-R interval • Wide QRS complex • Appearance of Delta wave
Ebstein Anomaly	**Hypothyroidism**	**Asd (Secundum Type)**
• RAH • RBBB	• Low voltage ECG • Flat or inverted T-wave	• RAD • RVH • RBBB • 1st degree AV block

Classification of Congenital Heart Diseases Based on ECG and CXR

Right Ventricular Hypertrophy

Cyanotic Defects

Decreased pulmonary blood flow

- Tetralogy of fallot
- TGA with pulmonary stenosis
- Eisenmenger syndrome

Increased pulmonary blood flow

- Aortic atresia
- Hypoplastic left heart syndrome
- TGA

Acyanotic Defects

- All left to right shunt defects with increase pulmonary vascular resistance
- Pulmonary stenosis

Left Ventricular Hypertrophy

Cyanotic Defects

Decreased pulmonary flow

- Tricuspid atresia

Increased pulmonary flow

- Single ventricle
- TGA with tricuspid atresia

Acyanotic Defects

- VSD
- PDA
- Septum premium ASD with mitral regurgitation
- Aortic stenosis
- Aortic regurgitation
- Coarctation of aorta
- Endocardial fibroelastosis
- Mitral regurgitation

Combined Ventricular Hypertrophy

Cyanotic Defects

Decreased pulmonary blood flow

- Single ventricle with pulmonary stenosis
- TGA

Increase Pulmonary blood flow

- TGA with pulmonary hypertension
- Single ventricle
- Truncus arteriosus
- VSD with moderate pulmonary stenosis

Acyanotic Defects

Left to right shunt

- Large VSD
- Large ASD
- Endocardial cushion defect

No Shunt

Pulmonary stenosis with aortic stenosis

CHAPTER 18

Outlines of Chest Roentogenography

- Quality
- Posture
- Chest Wall
- Diaphragm
- Mediastinum
- Hilar Shadow
- Lung Field

Outlines of Chest Roentogenography

Quality

The ribs and spine behind the heart can be identified when the lungs are not over exposed.

Posture

Medial ends of the clavicles are equidistant from the pedicle of vertebrae.

Chest Wall

Look for soft tissue swelling and ribs abnormality. Common causes of rib notching are coarctation of aorta, blalock taussig operation, venous fistula, neurofibromatosis and idiopathic.

Diaphragm

Right hemidiaphragm is at the level of anterior end of sixth rib. Left hemidiphragm is 2.5 cm lower. It is abnormal in abdominal distension, lung disease, subphernic abscess and phrenic nerve palsy.

Mediastinum

Check the mediastinal size and shifting. The common causes of enlarge mediastinum are:

- Retrosternal goiter
- Lymphadenopathy
- Neurogenic tumour
- Normal thymus or thymoma
- Hiatus hernia (air-fluid level)

Hilar Shadow

It is composed of pulmonary vessels and lymph nodes. Enlargement of hilar shadows should be differentiated whether due to pulmonary vessels or enlarged lymph node. If it is due to pulmonary vessels, it is a branching nature, usually bilateral and associated with enlargement of main pulmonary artery and heart. While the lymph node enlargement is lobulated.

Following are the causes of enlarged lymph node

- Tuberculosis
- Leukaemia
- Lymphoma
- Fungal infection

Lung Field

Check the Following Signs

- Silhouette sign
- Air bronchogram
- Sign of collapse
- Consolidation
- Spherical, linear and small widespread shadows
- Obstructive element
- Signs of pleural disease

Silhouette Sign

Obliterated border of aorta, heart or diaphragm is called silhouette sign. Loss of right upper border indicate lesion in anterior segment of upper lobe of right lung, similarly loss of right lower border indicate lesion in middle lobe. The lesion in lingular and anterior segment of upper lobe of left lung obliterate lower and upper left border of the heart respectively.

Air Bronchogram:

Visualization of air in intrapulmonary bronchi. Its presence indicates that lesion is always pulmonary. It is crowded in collapse and dilated in bronchiaetasis.

Consolidation (Table 17.1)

Following are the signs of consolidation.

1. Opaque shadow with ill defined borders
2. Air bronchogram
3. Silhouette sign

Sign of Collapse (Table17.2)

Following are the signs of collapse

1. Shadow of collapsed lobe
2. Silhouette sign
3. Hilar and Mediastinal pull
4. Crowding of bronchovascular markings
5. Narrowing of ribs
6. Elevation of diaphragm
7. Compensatory emphysema

Spherical, Linear, and Small Widespread Shadows (Table 17.3) Obstructive Element

Usually seen in obstructive lung disease like asthma, bronchiolitis, emphysema, cystic fibrosis, or meconium aspiration syndrome. Signs of obstructive element are:

1. Increase lung volume
2. Low and flat diaphragm
3. Elongated and narrowed heart
4. Attenuation of vessels

Signs of Pleural Disease

The two most common pleural pathologies are pleural effusion and pneumothorax. The former is presents as homogeneous opacity obliterating the costophrenic angles, lies outside the lung edge and higher laterally than medially. The diagnosis of Pneumothorax depends on recognizing pleural lines forming lung edge separated from chest wall, mediastinum or diaphragm by air, absence of vessels outside these lines, mediastinal shift and flattening of diaphragm. The causes of plueral effusion and pneumothorax are described in table 17.4 and 17.5 respectively.

Table 17.1   Causes of patchy consolidation/cavitation

Patchy Consolidation	Cavitation
• Infection	• Staphylococci
• Infraction	• Klebsiella
• Contusion	• Tuberculosis
• Immunological disorder	• Anaerobic Bacteria

Table 17.2   Causes of collapse

• Bronchial obstruction	• Bronchiectasis
• Pneumothorax	• Pulmonary embolus
• Pleural effusion	• Fibrosis of lobe

Table 17.3 Causes of spherical, linear and small widespread shadows

Spherical Shadows	Linear Shadows	Small Widespread Shadows
• Tuberculoma • Fungal granuloma • Metastasis • Lung Abscess • Calcification	• Septal lines • Pleuropulmonary scar • Pleural edge in pneumothorax • Emphysematous blebs	• Miliary tuberculosis • Sarcoidosis • Pulmonary oedema • Fibrosing alveolitis

Table 17.4 Causes of pleural effusion

• Subphernic abscess	• Nephrotic syndrome
• Cardiac failure	• Renal failure
• Pulmonary infarction	• Pneumonias

Table 17.5: Causes of pneumothorax

• Trauma	• Tuberculosis
• Emphysema	• Pneumonias

Table 17.6 Radiological findings of bronchiectasis

- Visible dilated bronchi
- Tubular or ring shadows containing air-fluid levels
- Persistent consolidation
- Loss of lung volume

Table 17.7 Difference between Hyaline Membrane Disease (HMD) and Meconium Aspiration Syndrome (MAS)

HMD	MAS
Widespread very small opacities	Usually patchy and Streaky
Visible air bronchograms	Less obvious air bronchogram
Uniform in distribution	Localised
No obstructive element	Diaphragm is low due to airway obstruction

'My doctor gave me six months to live, but when I could't pay the bill he gave me six months more.'

Walter Matthau

Vaccination

Immunization

The greatest achievement of past century in public health is immunization. Through routine vaccination children can now receive and be protected against approximately 16 different diseases. In developed countries annual incidence of diphtheria, paralytic poliomyelitis, measles, mumps, rubella, tuberculosis and fit, influenza type B have fallen more than 99%, while in third world and developing countries where routine vaccination is weak, incidence is still very high.

Immunization is a process by which specific protection against damaging pathogens is provided. Immunity is achieved by three means.

Active Immunization

Produced by the body following exposure to antigen.

Passive Immunization

Acquired by challenging the immune system with antibodies.

Herd Immunization

When a community is immunized for specific disease and coverage is >95% than the remaining population immunized by itself and protected.

Following are the general principles of immunization and recommended vaccine schedules Intra-dermal vaccine is given by 270 3/8 solo shot syringe at 30 degree of angle mainly on right deltoid for example BCG vaccine dose is 0.05 ml for infants . If the child is >1year (or for diagnostic BCG) then dose will be 0.1 ml s/c. Intra-muscular injection given at 90 degree angle to skin, with proper size and gauge of needle according to the age of baby to prevent the injuries to underlying nerves, blood vessels or bones. The anterolateral surface at the junction of upper 1/3 and lower 2/3 of thigh is the preferred site of vaccination in newborn and children up to 2 years of age. While deltoid muscle at upper outer quadrant is the preferred site of vaccination in children from 3 to18 years of age. Needle length and site of vaccination should be as follows:

NEWBORN 5/8 inch in thigh.

INFANTS (1 month–1 year) 1 inch in thigh CHLIDREN 1 year–18 years 1 1/4 inch in deltoid.

Type of Vaccines

Vaccines are of following types:

Bacterial

- Live e.g. BCG
- Dead e.g. Pertussis, Typhoid, Cholera
- Polyvalent e.g. Pneumococcal, Meningococcal

Viral

- Live e.g. OPV, measles, MMR
- Dead e.g. Rabies

Genetically Engineered

- Hepatitis 'B' vaccine
- HiB vaccine

Vaccination Schedule–EPI (Expanded Programme of Immunization)

Name of Vaccine	Age	Dose	Route
• BCG	At birth	0.05 ml	Intradermal
• OPV	At birth, 6 week, 10 week and 14 week.	1–2 drop	Oral
• DPT • Hep 'B' • Hib • Pneumococal	6 week, 10 week and 14 week.	0.5 cc	Intramuscular
• Measles	9 month	0.5 cc	Subcutaneous

Vaccination Schedule At Different Age Groups

Children Less Than 1 Year

- At birth   BCG and OPV0
- 6 weeks   Hep.B, DPT and OPV1, Hib, IPV
- 10 weeks   Hep.B, DPT and OPV2, Hib, IPV
- 14 weeks   Hep.B, DPT and OPV3, Hib, IPV
- At 9 months Measles

Children Less Than 2 Years

- BCG and measles
- Hep.B, DPT/OPV-3 doses at 4–8 week interval
- Booster of DPT and OPV after 1 year
- IPV-two doses at 2 months interval

Children 2–5 Year of Age

- BCG and measles (up to 4 years)
- DT/OPV-2 doses at 4–8 weeks interval
- Booster of DT and OPV after 1 year
- Hepatitis 'B' as above

Children After 5 Years

- BCG
- DT-2 doses at 4–8 weeks interval
- Hepatitis 'B' as above
  - Acute febrile illness is deferred to vaccination.
  - PCM, ARI, Gastroenteritis and moderate fever are not contraindications to vaccination.
  - Hospitalized children may receive the necessary vaccinations before discharge.

Vaccinations–Non EPI

Name	Dose	Interval	Route
Rota virus Vaccine	1–2 drop	< 6 months, at 2, 4 and 6 months. Booster at 15 months. > 6 months, two doses at 4 to 8 weeks interval, booster at 15 months > 1 year, two doses at 4 to 8 weeks interval > 15 months, single dose	PO
MMR	0.5 cc	Single dose at 12 months Booster at 5 years	I/M or S/C
Typhoid	0.5 cc	Single dose >2 years repeat after 3 years	I/M
Rabies	1 cc	Pre-exposure 0,7 and 28 days Post-exposure 0, 3, 7, 14, 28 days	I/M
Meningococcal	0.5 cc	Single dose	S/C or I/M
Chickenpox Vaccine	0.5 cc	9 months-12 years-1 dose > 13 years -2 doses at 6 -10 week interval	S/C
Hep 'A'		12 months, Booster at 18 months	
Flu vaccine	6 month 3 years 0.25 cc after 3 years 0.5 cc,	yearly	I/M

CHAPTER 20

Paediatric Procedures

- Blood Sampling and Cannulation
- Capillary Samples
- Intra Osseous Access
- Lumber Puncture
- Suprapubic Aspiration of Urine
- Umbilical Vein Catheterisation
- Radial Arterial Cannulation
- Endotracheal Intubation
- Chest Drains

Paediatric Procedures

Blood Sampling and Cannulation

Method

- Select the site for sampling. The following are the commonly used sites: back of hand/foot, antecubital fossa. Less common sites are ventral wrist, forearm, and scalp.

- Apply gentle traction to the skin from above to keep the vein position constant.

- Wipe with an alcohol swab

- Introduce the cannula at an angle of 45° through the skin and into the vein (Figure 20.2a). Flashback (blood visible in the hub of the needle) may not occur in small veins. If the vein was not entered, pull back (but not out), recheck the position and advance in a different line.

- Once in the vein, reduce the angle and go a very small way along the vein.

- While holding the needle still, advance the cannula over the needle and into the vein–usually carried out in one movement using the index finger of the same hand (Figure 20.2b). Blood may flow up the cannula (secondary flashback).

- Remove the needle and dispose it in a 'sharps' container.

- Sample blood with a syringe, then attach a T-piece or other appropriate connector and flush with 0.9% sodium chloride.

- Secure the cannula firmly. A splint may be required if it is near a joint.

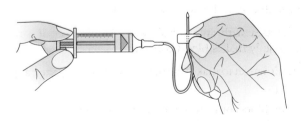

Fig. 20.1   Butterfly attached with syringe.

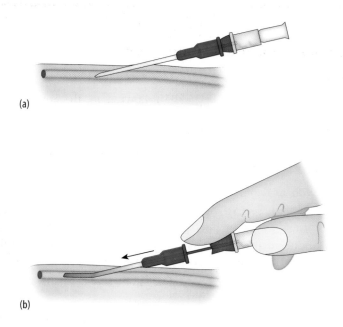

(a)

(b)

Fig. 20.2   Insertion of venous cannula.

Capillary Samples

Procedure

- Make sure the extremity is warm.

- In babies, use the sides of the heels (Figure 20.3). In older children the side of the thumb or big toe can be used.

- Clean the area with an alcohol swab. Application of a thin layer of petroleum jelly makes blood collection easier.

- Use a sterile lancet to make two punctures close together, approximately 2 mm deep.

- Collect the blood onto reagent strips or capillary tubes. Blood can be allowed to drip into bottles but venepuncture samples are preferred.

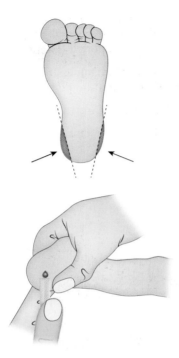

Fig. 20.3   Sites and technique for capillary blood sampling.

Intra Osseous Access

Procedure

This is an emergency procedure, contraindicated in long bone fracture in the same leg.

- Use an intraosseous or if unavailable, a bone marrow needle.

- The site used is the flat anterior surface of the tibia, a finger's breadth below and medial to the tibial tuberosity. Clean with an alcohol swab.

- Consider local anaesthetic if the child is conscious and there is time.

- Support the leg on a rolled up towel. Do not put fingers behind the limb in the path of the advancing needle.

- Firmly insert the needle using a turning or boring motion. There is a sudden 'give' when the needle enters the bone marrow. The needle should then stay upright unsupported (Figure 20.4).

- Remove the stylet and flush with saline. If there is swelling, the needle is not in the correct position and should be removed.

- Secure the needle. Any drug or fluid may be given by this route.

- Complications include: tibial fracture, osteomyelitis, compartment syndrome and skin necrosis.

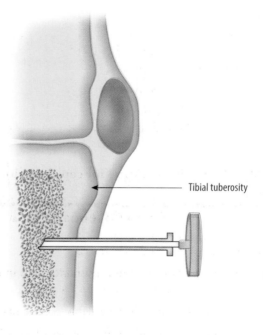

Tibial tuberosity

Fig. 20.4   Position of intraosseous needle for emergency vascular access.

Lumber Puncture (LP)

Contraindications

- Unstable child
- Platelet count less than 50,000
- Signs of raised intracranial pressure
- Reduced level of consciousness.

Procedure

- The child should be in the left lateral position and the lumbar spine should be as flexed as possible, with the plane of the back perpendicular to the bed. The assistant should hold the shoulders and behind the knees, rather than flex the neck.

- Clean the skin with antiseptic.

- The landmark is the top of the anterior superior iliac spine. A vertical line downwards leads to L3–4 or L4–5 spaces (Figure 20.5). Both are suitable.

- Hold the needle bevel upwards and pass it between the vertebral bodies aiming towards the umbilicus. Keep the needle horizontal. There is moderate resistance through the ligaments and then a 'give' as it passes into the CSF space.

- Remove the stylet-if pressure measurement is needed, connect the manometer and record the pressure.

- Drip the CSF into sterile pots and a fluoride bottle (for glucose), with 6 drops in each. Remove the needle and dress the site.

- The serum glucose should be measured at the time of the lumbar puncture to enable comparison between serum and CSF glucose.

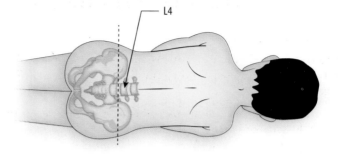

Fig. 20.5   Position and site for lumbar puncture.

Suprapubic Aspiration of Urine

Procedure

- Clean the suprapubic area with antiseptic solution.

- With an assistant holding the baby's legs, insert a 21G needle on a 10 ml syringe a finger's breadth above the symphysis pubis. Advance slowly, applying gentle suction with the syringe until urine appears (Figure 20.6).

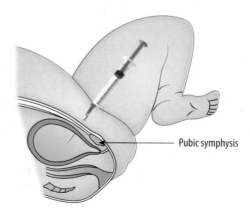

Fig. 20.6   Suprapubic aspiration.

Umbilical Vein Catheterisation

Procedure

A newborn baby has easily accessible umbilical vessels. Usually two arteries and one vein are present in the umbilical cord (Figure 20.7). The vein is large and may ooze blood.

- Calculate the distance to insert the line using a formula (weight (kg) x 3) + 4 cms or chart.

- Prepare and drape the patient.

- Flush the line with 0.9% saline and leave the syringe on the end.

- Wrap a tie loosely around the base then cut the cord down to 2–3 cm.

- Holding the cord with the forceps, identify the vein and insert the catheter to the calculated length.

- Secure the line by taping it to stitches through the cord. Do not apply tape directly on to the baby's fragile skin. Make sure it is secure.

- Check the position with a chest and abdominal X-ray.

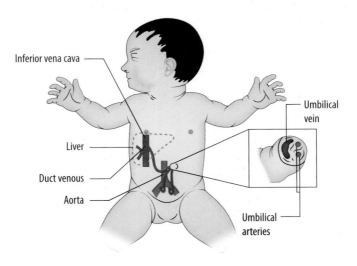

Fig. 20.7   Normal Anatomy of the umbilical cord.

Radial Arterial Cannulation

Procedure

- Palpate radial artery and support the wrist slightly extended for the radial artery (Figure 20.8).

- Find the pulse and insert the cannula towards it. The angle is shallower than for venous cannulation. Flashback will be pulsatile. Advance the cannula and remove the needle.

- If the artery is punctured but the catheter will not advance, remove it and apply firm pressure for 5 minutes.

- If there are any signs of ischaemia remove the cannula.

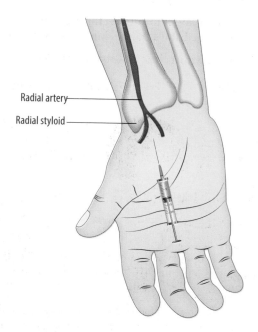

Fig. 20.8   Anatomy of radial artery.

Endotracheal Intubation

Requirements

- Non-sterile gloves
- Monitoring of oxygen saturation and heart rate
- Bag-valve-mask with oxygen supply
- Suction
- Laryngoscope (and spare) with a bright light and different -sized blades
- Suitably sized endotracheal (ET) tube plus one size above and below
- Tube size in children can be calculated using the formula Age/4 + 4 and tube length from Age /2 + 12. Term newborn.
- A means of securing the tube.
- A stethoscope.

Procedure

Infants need a tube size of 3.5. Premature infants will need a 3.0 or even a 2.5 sized tube.

Monitor oxygen saturation and heart rate during the procedure. Stop if it is not tolerated. A struggling child will require sedation and/or paralysis before intubation. An anaesthetist should normally supervise this in an older infant or child.

- Pre-oxygenate with bag-valve-mask ventilation
- A neonate needs a neutral head position; for older children extend the neck ('sniffing position')
- With the laryngoscope in the left hand, introduce the blade in the right side of the mouth and centralise, moving the tongue out of the way (see Figure 20.9a).
- Insert the laryngoscope blade down to the vallecula before the epiglottis (Figure 20.9a). In babies it is easier to go into the oesophagus and pull back until the cords appear (Figure 20.9b). Be careful not to traumatize the larynx.

- Pressure on the cricoid helps bring the cords into view-use the little finger of the left hand or ask a helper to do it.

- Gently suction out secretions.

- Insert the ET tube and stop once the black mark (near the tip) is past the cords.

Note the length at the lips. Do not insert the ET tube if the cords cannot be seen. Do not push against closed cords.

- Once the ET tube is in, listen to air entry (while bagging) in both axillae and over the stomach. Louder sounds on the right indicate the tube is in the right main bronchus: pull it back slightly and listen again. If the sounds are loudest over the stomach with little chest expansion then the tube is in the oesophagus: remove it.

- Secure the ET tube and confirm position with a chest X-ray.

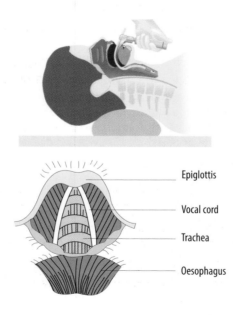

Epiglottis

Vocal cord

Trachea

Oesophagus

Fig. 20.9 Endotracheal intubation: (a) laryngoscope position; (b) view of vocal cords

Chest Drains

Procedure

- Support the child with the affected side up.

- Aim for the 4th or 5th intercostal space in the mid-axillary line. The position should be guided by ultrasound in empyema.

- Infiltrate local anaesthetic.

- Make an incision just above and parallel with the rib, avoiding the intercostal vessels and nerve that lie inferior to each rib (Figure 20.10). With fine forceps bluntly dissect down to the pleura.

- Do not use the trocar in the chest drain–use the forceps to insert it. After initial resistance it will pop through the pleura. Advance it so all the holes are inside the chest.

- Connect the drain to the seal/valve. Stitch the incision closed. Secure the tube with a stitch and use an occlusive dressing over the whole site.

- Confirm drain position with a chest X-ray.

- If the drain is not bubbling, applying a small amount of suction may help.

- The drain can be removed once it has stopped bubbling for 24 hours. Remove it on expiration (crying). Close the incision and perform a CXR after 2–4 hours.

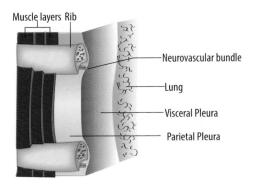

Fig. 20.10 Anatomy of the chest wall for chest drain insertion.

CHAPTER 21

Normal Values and Paediatric Formulas

- Weight
- Height
- OFC
- Surface Area
- Blood Pressure
- ETT-size
- Fluid Requirement
- Caloric Requirement
- Normal Blood Values
- Base Deficit
- Respiratory Rate
- Heart Rate

Normal Values and Paediatric Formulas

Weight

Weight (3–12 months) = $\dfrac{\text{Age (month)} + 9}{2}$

Weight (1–6 years) = Age (year) x 2 +8

Weight (7–12 year) = $\dfrac{\text{Age (year)} \times 7 - 5}{2}$

Height

Height (2–12year) = Age (year) x 6 + 77

OFC

OFC (Up to 1 year) = $\dfrac{\text{Length (cms)} + 9.5}{2}$

Surface Area

Surface area (m2) =

Weight (kg) x 4 + 7/ Weight (kg) + 90

Median Blood Pressure

Median blood pressure (systolic) = Age (years) x 2+90

Endotracheal Tube Size

Endotracheal tube size = (Age in years. + 16)/4

Fluid Requirements

1st10 Kg–100 cc/kg/day

11–20 Kg–50 cc/kg/day

21– onward–20 cc/kg/day

OR 1500 cc/m2/day

Caloric Requirements

1st10 Kg–100cal/kg/day

11–20 Kg–50cal/kg/day

21– onward–20cal/kg/day

Normal Blood Values (Means with Ranges)

Age	Hb (g%)	TLC Per mm3	Neu (%)	Lymphos (%)
Birth	17	18	60	32
	(14–20)	(9–30)	(40–80)	
6–weeks.	17	12	40	48
	(13–20)	(5–21)	(30–50)	
6 months-6 years	12	10	42	51
	(10.5–14)	(6–15)	(32–52)	
12 years	14	7.5	60	30
	(12–16)	(5–10)	(40–75)	(20–45)

Base Deficit

Sodium	weight	x deficit x 0.3
Potasium	weight	x deficit x 0.6
Bicarbonate	weight	x deficit x 0.3

Respiratory Rate

Age	Range of Tachypnea
< 2 months	> 60 breaths/ minute
2 months to 1 year	> 50 breaths/ minute
1 to 3 years	> 40 breaths/ minute
3 to 5 years	> 30 breaths/ minute

Heart Rate

Mean foetal heart rate is 140 beats/minute, reduces 10 beats/minute by every age group.

Age Group	Heart Rate (mean)
Foetus	140
Neonate (up to 1 month)	130
Infant (up to 1 year)	120
Toddler (1–3 years)	110
Preschool age (3–5 years)	100
Early School age (5–10 years)	90
Late School age (10–15 years)	80
Adult	70

'A drug is that substance which, when injected into a rat, will produce a scientific report.'

Anonymous

CHAPTER 22

Common Definitions

- Perinatal
- Growth
- Genetic/Dysmorphology
- Neurological
- Respiratory
- Dermatological
- Genito-Urinary
- Gastrointestinal
- Ear, Nose and Throat
- Visual
- Orthopedic

Common Definitions

PERINATAL

Abortion	Product of conception born dead before 24 weeks gestation.
Birth rate	Number of births per 1000 population.
Embryo	The human conceptus for the first 10 weeks after conception(and in practise for the first 12 weeks measured from the first day of the mother's last menstrual period.
Extreme low birth weight	Weighing less than or equal to 1000g at the time of birth.
Extreme preterm	Gestation less than 28 completed weeks measured from the first day of mother's last menstrual period.
Foetus	The human conceptus after the embryonic phase until the moment of delivery.
Hydramnios	Excessive amount of amniotic fluid.
Infant mortality rate	Number of deaths in the first year of life per 1000 live births.
Low birth weight	Weighing less than or equal to 2500 g at the time of birth.
Neonatal mortality rate	Number of deaths in the first month of life per 1000 live births.
Oligohydramnios	Diminished volume of amniotic fluid.
Perinatal mortality rate	Number of stillbirths and first week neonatal deaths per 1000 live births.
Polyhydramnios	Excessive amount of amniotic fluid.

Post-term	Gestation greater than 42 weeks measured from the first day of mother's last menstrual period.
Preterm	Gestation less than 37 completed weeks measured from the first day of mother's last menstrual period.
Small for gestational age	Birth weight less than the tenth centile for a given gestation.
Stillbirth	Child born dead after 24 weeks of gestation.
Term	Gestation 37 completed weeks to 42 completed weeks after the first day of mother's last menstrual period.
Very low birth weight	Weighing less than or equal to 1500g at the time of birth.

GROWTH

Failure to thrive	Inadequate growth velocity.
Height velocity	Centimetres increase in 1 year at that age (quote as centile).
Weight velocity	Kilograms increase in 1 year at that age (quote as centile).

GENETIC/DYSMORPHOLOGY

Arachnodactyly	Long slender (spider) digits.
Camptodactyly	Permanent flexion of an interphalangeal joint usually of the first finger.
Clinodactyly	Permanent deflexion of one or more fingers.
Congenital	Present at the time of birth.

Consanguinity	Related by blood (usually of related parents, e.g. first cousins).
Dysmorphism	Having unusual physical features (e.g. low set ears, syndactyly).
Cryptorchidism	Failure of descent of the testes.
Glossoptosis	Downward displacement of the tongue.
Hypomandibularism	Smallness of the mandible.
Micrognathia	Smallness of the mandible.
Phocomelia	Flipper limb (e.g. seen after thalidomide teratogenesis).
Polydactyly	The presense of more than five digits on a hand or foot.
Ranula	Sublingual cyst.
Syndactyly	The joining together of two or more fingers or toes.
Syndrome	A pattern of unusual features. (e.g. Down's or cri-du-chat).
Teratogenic	Causing embryonic or foetal abnormality.

NEUROLOGICAL

Ataxia	A loss of motor coordination.
Athetosis	A condition of constant involuntary slow writhing movements.
Cerebral palsy	A motor disorder resulting from a non-progressive lesion of the developing region.
Diplegia	A type of cerebral palsy with symmetrical paresis of the limb, especially the lower limbs and usually with rigidity or spasticity.

Dysarthria	Difficulty in coordinating speech.
Dysdiadochokinesis	Difficulty in performing rapid alternating movements.
Dyskinesis	Difficulty with voluntary movements.
Dysmetria	Difficulty judging distance.
Hemiparesis	Partial paralysis of one side of the body.
Hemiplegia	Paralysis of one side of the body.
Myalgia	Muscle pain.
Quadriplegia	Paralysis affecting all four limbs.
Syncope	Fainting.

RESPIRATORY

Dyspnea	Difficulty in breathing.
Hyperpnoea	Overbreathing.
Orthopnea	Difficulty with breathing except when erect (either standing or sitting).
Pectus carinatum	Pigeon chest (prominent sternum).
Pectus excavatum	Hollow chest (sternal depression).
Stridor	A sound predominantly inspiratory in character, resulting from the rapid passage of air through a partially obstructed larynx or trachea.
Tachypnea	Rapid respiration.
Wheeze	A musical sound, predominantly expiratory in character, resulting from the rapid passage of air through partially obstructed bronchi.

DERMATOLOGICAL

Alopecia	Baldness.
Blister	An elevated serum-filled lesion.
Bruise	Bleeding into the subcutaneous tissues.
Bulla	A large blister.
Ecchymosis	A purple area caused by extravasation of blood into the skin.
Exanthema	A skin eruption as a symptom of a general disease (e.g. measles).
Haemangioma	A vascular lesion, usually congenital.
Ichthyosis	Dry scaly skin.
Impetigo	A pustular skin rash caused by staphylococci or streptococci.
Lentigo	A brown macule, like a freckle with a regular border.
Macule	A circumscribed non-palpable discolouration of the skin.
Morbilliform	Measle-like.
Naevus	A vascular, pigmented or hairy skin lesion, usually congenital.
Papule	A small raised palpable lesion.
Petechiae	Pinhead purpura.
Pruritus	Itchiness.
Purpura	Multiple spontaneous haemorrhages into the skin or mucous membranes.
Pustule	An elevated pus-containing lesion.
Seborrhoea	Overaction of the sebaceous glands.
Telangiectasia	Localised capillary dilation.

Urticaria (hives, nettle rash)	An eruption of itching wheals.
Varicelliform	Chickenpox-like.
Verruca	A wart.
Vesicle	A blister 0.5 cm or less in diameter.
Vitiligo	A condition of skin depigmentation.
Wheal	An urticarial eruption: A pink or white raised area surrounded by a flare of erythema.

GENITO-URINARY

Balanitis	Inflammation of the foreskin.
Chordee	Ventral angulation of the shaft of the penis.
Enuresis	Involuntary passage of urine, usually used of bed wetting.
Epispadias	With the urethral orifice emerging on the dorsum of the penis.
Hydrocoele	A collection of serous fluid in the tunica vaginalis of the scrotum.
Hypospadias	With the urethral orifice emerging on the undersurface of the penis.

GASTROINTESTINAL

Atresia	Congenital absence of an opening, passage or cavity, especially with reference to complete bowel blockage due to failure of development of the lumen.
Bulimia	Morbidly increased appetite often alternating with periods of anorexia.

Encopresis	Involuntary passage of faeces.
Intussusception	The infolding of one segment of the intestine with another.
Scaphoid	Hollowed out.
Stenosis	Narrowing.

EAR, NOSE AND THROAT

Epistaxis	Nose bleeding.
Glue ear	Serous otitis media.

VISUAL

Amblyopia	Partial loss of sight.
Aniridia	Absence of the iris.
Aphakia	Absence of the crystalline lens.
Chalazion	A chronic inflammatory granuloma of the eyelid.
Coloboma	A congenital cleft of the iris.
Hordeolum	Stye.
Hyphema	Blood in the anterior chamber of the eye.
Strabismus	A squint.
Uveitis	Inflammation of the iris, ciliary body and choroid.

ORTHOPEDIC

Genu recurvatum	A condition of hyperextension of the knee.
Genu valgum	Knock-kneed.
Genu varum	Bow-legged.
Gibbus	Extreme kyphosis with a sharply angulated segment.
Kyphosis	An abnormal curvature of the spine with convexity backwards.
Osteomyelitis	Inflammation of the bone marrow and adjacent bone.
Osteoporosis	Marbling of the bones leading to obliteration of the marrow.
Scoliosis	Lateral curvature of the spine.
Talipes calaneovalgus	Club foot with dorsal flexion (i.e. heel on ground) and eversion.
Talipes equinovarus	Club foot, with extension and inversion at the ankle.

'A good marriage would be between a blind wife and a deaf husband.'

Michel de Montaigne

CHAPTER 23

Common Investigations

- Complete Blood Count
- Arterial Blood Gases-ABG
- Urea, Creatinine and Electrolytes-UCE
- Urine Detail Report-D/R

Complete Blood Count

Haemoglobin

- High at birth (18 g/dl)

- Lowest at 2 months (range 8.5 -14 g/dl).

- Low haemoglobin indicates anaemia.

Mean Cell Volume (MCV)

- Microcytic anaemia (MCV < 76 fl) is usually due to iron deficiency, thalassaemia trait or lead poisoning.

- Macrocytosis (MCV > 100fl) may reflect folate or B12 deficiency.

White Blood Cells

- Leucocytosis usually reflects infection–neutrophilia and left shift (i.e. immature neutrophils) implies bacterial infection.

- Lymphocytosis is more common in viral infections, atypical bacterial infection and whooping cough.

- Neutropenia (neutrophils <1.0 x 109/l) can occur in severe infection or due to immunosuppression.

Platelets

- High platelet count usually reflects bleeding, iron defeciency or inflammation (e.g. Kawasaki disease).

- Low platelet count is commonly seen with idiopathic thrombocytopenic purpura (ITP) and infection.

- Platelets are functionally abnormal (e.g. von Willebrand disease, or rarely Glanzmann disease or Bernard Soulier disease).

Peripheral Film

There may be poikilocytes (iron defeceincy), target cell(thalesemia), acanthocyte (abetalipoproteinemia), blast cell (leukaemia) or spherocyte (H.spherocytosis).

Arterial Blood Gases-ABG

Normal arterial blood gas values

PH	7.35–7.42
PCO2	4.0–5.5 kPa
PO2	11–14 kPa (children) 8–10 (neonatal period)
HCO3–	17–27 mmol/l

Determining the type of blood gas abnormality

	PH	PCO2	PO2	HCO3
Metabolic	Low	N	N	Low
Respiratory acidosis	Low	High	N/low	N
Metabolic alkalosis	High	N	N	High
Respiratory alkalosis	High	Low	N/ High	N
Compensated respiratory acidosis	N	High	N	High

Metabolic Acidosis

- Severe gastroenteritis.
- Perinatal asphyxia (build up of lactic acid).
- Shock.

- Diabetic ketoacidosis.

- Inborn errors of metabolism.

- Loss of bicarbonate (renal tubular acidosis).

Respiratory Acidosis

Respiratory failure and underventilation.

Metabolic Alkalosis

Usually due to vomiting e.g. pyloric stenosis.

Respiratory Alkalosis

- Hyperventilation (e.g. anxiety).

- Salicylate poisoning: causes initial hyperventilation and then metabolic acidosis due to acid load).

Urea, Creatinine and Electrolytes-UCE

Normal ranges

Sodium	135–145 mmol/l
Potassium	3.5–5.0 mmol/l
Chloride	96–110 mmol/l
Bicarbonate	17–27 mmol/l
Creatinine	20–80 mmol/l
Urea	2.5–6.5 mmol/l

Characteristic Patterns of UCE

Pyloric Stenosis

- Metabolic alkalosis

- Low chloride

- Low potassium concentration (due to repeated vomiting and loss of stomach acid) and a Low sodium concentration.

Diabetic Ketoacidosis

- Metabolic acidosis

- Low bicarbonate

- High potassium

- High urea and creatinine

Gastroenteritis

- Urea concentration is high

- Sodium may be either high or low

Hypernatraemia (Na+ > 145 mmo/l)

- Dehydration–fluid deprivation or diarrhoea

- Excessive sodium intake

Hyponatraemia (Na<135 mmol/l)

- Sodium loss
  - Diarrhoea (especially if replacement fluids hypotonic)
  - Renal loss (renal failure)
  - Cystic fibrosis (loss in sweat)

- Water excess:
  - ○ Excessive intravenous fluid administration
  - ○ SIADH (inappropriate antidiuretic hormone secretion)

Hyperkaleamia (<5.5 mmol/l)

- Acute renal failure
- Massive haemolysis or tissue necrosis.
- Congenital adrenal hyperplasia.

Hypokalaemia (<3.5 mol/l)

- Diarrhoea and vomiting
- Diuretic therapy
- Inadequate intake (e.g. starvation)

Urine Detail Report-D/R

Colour

Dark Yellow

- Concentrated urine
- Bile pigments

Red Colour

- Blood
- Myoglobin
- Porphyrin
- Red food colours

Dark Brown or Black

- Homogentasic acid
- Blood

PH

Acidic in renal tubular acidosis

RBCs Positive

- Glomerular disease(e.g. AGN)
- UTI
- Bleeding disorder
- Stone
- Drugs
- Exercise

Pus Cell

UTI

Proteinuria

- False Traces/+ 30 mg/Dl
- ++ 100 mg/dL
- +++ 300 mg/dL
- ++++ 2000 mg/dL

Causes

- Postural
- Exercise

- Fever
- Tubular disease(e.g. Acute tubular necrosis)
- Glomerular disease(e.g. Nephrotic syndrome)

False Positive Proteinuria

- Highly concentrated urine
- pH >8.0
- Haematuria
- Contaminated with chlorhexidine

Sugar Positive

Diabetes Mellitus

Ketones in Urine

- Starvation
- High ketogenic diet
- Diabetic ketoacidosis

Index

H

I

J

K

L

O

P